THE
NEW FAST FOOD
CALORIE GUIDE

By
Marcia LaSota

GABRIEL BOOKS

Published by   GABRIEL BOOKS
                (A Division of Minnesota Scholarly Press)
                Mankato, Minnesota

Illustrated by Peter Demarest and Jeff Irish

Distributed by

        U.S.A. Independent Publishers Group
                One Pleasant Avenue
                Port Washington, N.Y. 11050

        Canada Fforbez Publications
                2133 Quebec St
                Vancouver, B.C.

ISBN 0-933474-33-4

TABLE OF CONTENTS

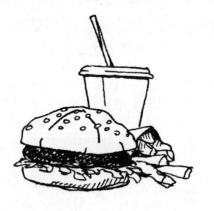

PREFACE

When the first edition of THE FAST FOOD CALORIE GUIDE was published in early 1980, calorie counts were dangerously high in most franchise outlets! The typical hamburger, cheeseburger, fish fillet, and slice of pizza carried a terrific clout of calories. At that time I warned consumers that just one meal at a fast food restaurant could provide more than half of all the calories needed for an entire day! And one meal, added to two others at home or another restaurant, would impose a significant weight gain on the average customer!

Thus it comes as a welcome surprise to discover that, in the most recent survey of fast food franchises, several restaurants have significantly lowered calorie counts of individual menu items. In particular two of the largest franchises, Hardee's and Kentucky Fried Chicken, are dramatically lower. Hardee's has

1

cut the amount of fat in a Big Deluxe almost in half, with a corresponding beneficial decrease in cholesterol. Kentucky Fried Chicken meals also are down significantly compared to the survey of two years ago!

With two major chains leading the way, I look for the rest of the industry to show much greater concern for the nutritional needs of its customers. Although there is continued worry about the small amounts of minerals and vitamins and for the large amounts of iodine and salt in some fast food meals, the evidence that fat, carbohydrates, and calories are of increasing concern is a healthy sign and I hope a trend that the entire fast food industry will participate in during coming years!

Marcia LaSota

INTRODUCTION

In the competitive beehive of the fast food industry, menus constantly change as franchises introduce fresh products and attempt to attract new customers. Also, formulas for preparation of individual menu items change from time to time, consequently affecting the caloric content of food items.

The menus listed in this guide for fast foods may not necessarily contain all the menu items offered by each restaurant, since the menus change so often, nor can the caloric value assigned to each menu remain constant as franchises change the composition of steak sandwiches, chicken, pizza, hamburgers, and other foods. But the guide does contain most of the current menus of major fast food restaurant chains and the information is as current as the

3

author was able to provide right up to press time. Future updated editions of the guide are projected to follow at regular intervals.

The first section of the book contains a brief history of the food industry and examines the success of fast food restaurants. Calories for food items in the major restaurants appear in this section.

The second section of the guide is for diabetics and provides complete diabetic food exchange values for many fast food outlets.

The third section is a summary of nutritional analyses of fast food, showing protein, carbohydrates, fat, sodium, and cholesterol levels among fast food meals.

SECTION

ONE

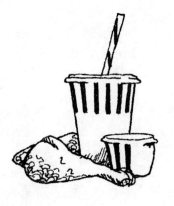

FAST FOOD — FAST CALORIES

The average American eats nearly half of all meals in restaurants and more and more of those meals are consumed at Burger King, A & W, McDonald's, Kentucky Fried Chicken, Hardee's, Tastee Freeze, Dairy Queen, Pizza Hut, Jack in the Box, and other fast food chains that sell more than ten billion dollars of food to the American public each year.

The astounding popularity of fast food restaurants seems to be tied to the manias of speed, security, and conformity in American society. And the first factor, speed, should not be taken lightly! The Frenchman's leisurely lunch of cheese, bread, and wine is as rare in America as kippers for breakfast. Twelve sharp, out of the delivery truck or office, into the line at the burger shop, no shocks at the cash register, safely away two minutes later to table, bench or car where a Big Mac, fries and shake can be wolfed down before going on to more important business or leisure activities. Rarely in America is luncheon a time for relaxed conversation and delight in simple but enjoyable food as is true in many other parts of the world.

As for the second factor, security, there are no surprises in the fast food trade. Any item can be ordered with the same shape and taste it possessed yesterday, or the day before or the day before that. Fast food is a repeat customer industry. People return time after time to order identical tasting food and identical sized portions. If, as one advertising executive remarked, "Your local burger joint is selling security, not hamburger," then the product must be something the American consumer values more than food because fast food restaurants do not offer distinctive food or good nutrition.

With some exceptions, food in fast food restaurants does offer the basic vitamins, proteins, and minerals to fulfill minimum daily allowances of these nutrients. But nutrient deficiencies are not the chief concern! The salient problem with menus in the fast food industry is the overabundance of calories and other agents like iodine that appear in far larger than necessary amounts in a typical fast food restaurant meal. Virtually all the tests of food in this industry proved far too rich in calories. In fact, many typical, single meals provide about one-half of all the calories needed for an entire day by a normal adult male, and far too many calories than needed by women and children. Just one of these fast food meals, added to two other daily meals at home or at other restaurants, would put significant added weight on the average male customer. The weight gain would be even more pronounced if the consumer was an office worker who ate his Big Mac or Whopper and then sat at a desk for the remainder of the day. A female office worker would gain even more weight because she needs fewer calories than the average male in order to maintain normal body weight.

Today, studies indicate that nearly half of all Americans are overweight. And young adults are at least twenty per-cent heavier than their parents were at a similar age. Young children are in even greater danger in the war with obesity. Oversalted, brightly packaged fast food meals are very popular with children of nearly all ages. Children are subjected to a barrage of television advertisements extolling the novelty of Ronald McDonald's latest product offering and a smorgasbord of other industry items. McDonald's is the largest advertiser in the industry. The Company spent more than 40 million dollars on advertising in 1979, advertising that has been so successful it prompted a competitor to claim "McDonald's hamburgers would taste good even if they left the meat out."

Other fast food chains are increasing the size of their advertising budgets after observing the success of McDonald's advertising blitz. Saturday morning television is one long gastronomic journey whose scenery includes but one green vegetable—Popeye's spinach. Surveys have shown how effective this advertising is in luring young children and their parents toward pizza, chicken, fish, and hamburger stands where far too often stomachs are deluged with too thick shakes, too much grease, and staggering amounts of calories.

Too large a percentage of fast food calories come in substances like sugar and other sweeteners that provide virtually no nutrition what-so-ever! Cola drinks, the favorite liquid ordered to wash down meals, are an enormously profitable item for retailers and an enormously unprofitable item (from a nutritional standpoint) for the customer. Cola beverages average more than 100 calories per drink yet they contain nothing of nutritional value. Milk shakes, misnamed because they rarely contain milk or ice cream, are almost as bad as cola drinks. These "shakes" actually are made from a mix of vegetable fats, artificial sweeteners and other flavors having more than twice as many calories as a glass of milk.

The beef used in most fast food hamburger chains has less fat content than the average ground chuck, but when mayonnaise and other sauces are added to burgers to, depending on your point of view, enhance or disguise their taste, the caloric content rises to undesirable levels.

In addition to an excess of calories, another disturbing quantity in fast food meals was reported in *Consumer Reports Magazine*, May,

11

1975. In its tests of fast foods, *Consumer Reports* discovered iodine in amounts averaging more than 30 times the Recommended Daily Allowance for this substance. The iodine apparently is contained in iodized salt, rolls, and breads or from residues of iodine compounds used to clean and sterilize food-processing equipment. Little is known of the effects of such high levels of iodine in food, but it is known that "too much iodine could affect the proper functioning of the thyroid gland."

Conversely, there are items necessary to good health that are in too short supply in fast food meals. Six of these nutrients most commonly in short supply are biotin, folacin, pantothenic acid, iron, copper and total vitamin A.

As for the myth that fast food meals are less expensive than home cooking, the November, 1975, issue of *Good Housekeeping* demolished that argument with a study showing that restaurant pizza can cost twice as much as home-made pizza, specialty burgers may be from twenty to forty cents more than home-made equivalents, and so on. In effect, fast food restaurants are selling another ideal dear to the minds but not pocketbooks or stomachs of

Americans, and that ideal is basically convenience.

Where will it all end? The United States may soon be saturated with fast food restaurants! The Department of Commerce says there are now more than 50,000 of them. Some have predicted that as the medium age continues to grow older customers may begin to drift away from the numbing sameness and colossal caloric content of fast food. But at the moment fast food franchises are as popular as TV dinners were for an earlier generation of Americans!

Chapter Two

CONVENIENCE, PROCESSED FOODS —FAST SUCCESS

How did fast food restaurants become as popular as they are today?

In a few short years, new techniques of preservation, freezing, and packaging, combined with new equipment like micro-wave ovens, revolutionized restaurant practices throughout the industry.

For eons man consumed foods that did not require cooking or other preparation. Nuts, fruit, some vegetables, and some seafood can be consumed raw. Simple preservation techniques like salting, smoking, and bread making have existed since the early civilizations of Egypt and Babylon. Canning and bottling, however, are far younger methods of preservation. A Frenchman discovered how to preserve foods by canning only in the late 18th century, and canneries rapidly spread through Europe and through America offering a remarkable variety of preserved foods: meats, macaroni, spaghetti, fish, pickles, jams, salads, soups, fruit, vegetables, and a king's banquet in cans, where only a short time before fresh foods formed the bulk of a typical family diet.

The shift from freshly butchered meats, fish, vegetables and other staples, to preserved and packaged grocery items was accelerated by the two world wars.

During the First World War, new techniques of preserving and packaging food were invented to supply American armies in Europe. In World War Two, new preservation techniques were coupled with a need to increase the speed of food service. Here was the birth of assembly line commissaries and other fast food processes. The Armed Services needed food production systems that did not require heavy labor. Food vending machines filled the need, and central commissaries supplied mass production food. These machines supplying precooked meals became more and more sophisticated and enormously popular with the general public following World War Two.

16

The popularity of convenience foods paralleled the successes of the vending industry. Clarence Birdseye had been tinkering with convenience products since the early 1920's. In a Gloucester, Massachusetts laboratory he packaged pre-cooked fruits, vegetables, meats and fish, and marketed them in New England under the Birdseye trade name. Success was elusive. Primitive home freezers, inadequate distribution, the Great Depression, a nation where electrification was still a novelty—all contributed to dampen enthusiasm for new methods of supplying foods.

However, after World War Two frozen orange juice concentrate was introduced and became an immediate success. Birdseye and other companies added dozens of frozen food items to stores and markets and the age of convenience foods was born! Frozen french fried potatoes were introduced in 1950 and soon rivaled orange juice in popularity. Swanson brought out chicken pot pies and chicken a la king. They became so popular, the concept was expanded to include complete dinners on aluminum trays. And since the dinners were marketed to appeal to viewers of television which also was enjoying sensational popularity with the American public, the precooked meals were appropriately called TV dinners!

In the early 1960's the plastics industry invented a pouch which protected food inside the package while it was immersed in boiling water. This technology was also applied to other new types of disposable packages. Tab pull cans and other aluminum containers, paper and foil combinations and varied plastic containers crowded onto display shelves. As more effective methods of preserving and freezing foods were combined with revolutionary packages and containers, virtually any type of food could be merchandised in precooked and frozen packages.

What had been a loose assortment of entrepreneurs and distributors like Birdseye and Swanson, grew with amazing rapidity into an enormously profitable industry! Networks of storage lockers and refrigerated trucks and boxcars were developed to transport the mountains of frozen foods. These easy-to-prepare convenience foods were devoured by American families with the enthusiasm of starving Indian peasants dipping into bags of free wheat. Shoppers discovered an enticing collection of newly packaged delights. Younger generations may take the astounding variety of precooked foods on grocery shelves for granted, but those who visited grocery markets regularly during the decades of the 1950's and 1960's remember how new frozen food items cropped up with the frequency of trinkets on dime store shelves and were snapped up just as eagerly by curious consumers.

With the success of pre-cooked dinners, frozen food processors and equipment manufacturers plowed large chunks of their swelling profits into advanced research to find more sophisticated methods of preparing and reconstituting convenience foods. This research yielded better high speed steam cookers, charbroilers, automatic deep fat fryers, convention ovens, more efficient freezers, and thawing refrigerators, and that pandora's box of the frozen food trade—the microwave oven. Preprepared foods, as they are now known in the trade, include an astounding number and variety of items. In the industry, a pre-prepared food is defined as anything that can be served with little or no preliminary preparation other than heating or cooling to increase palatability. This includes "fabricated and engineered," freeze dried, dehydrated and intermediate moisture food items, as well as canned, fermented, pickled, cured, sugar concentrated and convenience items. The food service industry categorizes all pre-prepared frozen items as convenience foods: vegetables, juices, beverages, fruits, meat, poultry, seafood, soups, pies, special dinners, snacks, desserts and bakery products. The fastest growing segment of this market is in precooked, frozen meats. Pastrami, corned beef, hamburger patties, shish kebab, spare ribs, main course dinners, pre-fabricated and pre-cooked veal patties, and pre-cooked meatballs are the favorites. Pre-cooked meatballs are used to prepare many dishes like pizzas, soups, and spaghetti, while pre-cooked hamburger can easily be heated without shrinkage and served in sports areas, schools, and other "volume feeding establishments" as they are known in the trade.

The enormous popularity of fast food and convenience menus has had an enormous and disquieting influence on other restaurants.

Precooked frozen food is now served in

luxury restaurants from San Francisco to New York. Where gourmet restaurants once prepared virtually everything from scratch, now they can purchase precooked, frozen Chicken Kiev, Cordon Bleu, Lobster Newburgh, and dozens of other "gourmet dishes" that are available from food processors and are served up routinely as original concoctions.

Some San Franciscans were so disturbed by the trend in precooked restaurant food, they proposed an ordinance to require labeling of frozen menu items by all restaurants, whose owners rallied in opposition and worked for its successful defeat.

Fewer cooks and chefs are needed with precooked menus! Food industry firms offer courses on "reconstituting convenience foods." Restaurants no longer have to seek out the freshest asparagus, or the choicest cuts of meats. They no longer need to stand in attentive supervision of food on the broiler. Preparation merely requires someone to stoke the microwave ovens and make sure the timers are set.

If diners do not notice the difference between fresh and frozen food, as the industry contends, then restauranters certainly can tell the difference in profits. Fast food joints routinely turn a 400 percent profit on a sack of french fries. Gourmet restaurants make equivalent profits on a pre-cooked and frozen Chicken Kiev purchased from a distributor for $2.00 and sold to the customer by candlelight for $8.00. Restaurants that took pride in the menus offered to customers once were happy to pay up to 50 percent of the customers' bill for fresh, outstanding produce. No longer!

Not only are profits growing at the expense of quality, but also many restaurants, ever greedy for more leverage, routinely take a day's supply of menu items out of the freezer and allow them to thaw to about 40 degrees before preparation in the oven. At closing time, any unordered items are returned to the freezer for a repeat performance, perhaps answering your curiosity about soggy, unappetizing messes that occasionally are presented with a proud flourish at your favorite restaurant.

By the middle of the 1970's, food industry magazines were reporting that more than half of surveyed restaurants reported using some

22

precooked frozen dinner items and were planning to use, much, much more.

Do consumers object to the taste of such foods? On the contrary, there is evidence that the American public has become so accustomed to pre-cooked, artificially flavored foods that natural products taste "funny" and are avoided! This is particularly true with vegetables, condiments like catsup, fruit juices, and other staples. It is true that a large minority prefers a "natural" diet with emphasis on granola, fresh fruits and vegetables, lean meats or a vegetarian diet, and other natural tasting, nutritious foods. But a far larger number of American consumers have come to accept processed food as the norm, and the taste of freshly harvested green beans from the garden—cooked minimum time and then savored for their rich, substantial taste by the home gardener—may in turn repel those who are used to a diet of frozen green beans from the supermarket, beans that are boiled until virtually all color and nutrients are destroyed, whereupon artificial flavorings and color are added so that in comparison to the fresh product, these beans are like eating a pair of mildewed socks.

There is a large and growing industry of food flavorists who perform research and advise companies on the marketing of products. The usual advice from such companies is to avoid trying to duplicate natural flavors in canned, powdered, concentrated, and freeze-dried foods. The metallic taste of many frozen fruit juices is more acceptable in the marketplace than the less sweet and pungent taste of freshly squeezed oranges. The average consumer would pass up a loaf of warm, fragrant homemade bread for a slice of Wonder Bread. Why? Because the tastebuds of the American public have been indoctrinated with imitation tastes which over the years have displaced the real with the artificial, so that artificial flavorings are finally perceived as natural—a marvel of modern advertising and merchandising!

And nowhere in the supermarket/food/ restaurant industries has success with processed products been more pronounced than in fast food franchises. They established the trend and capitalized fully on its potential with the American public, and also with European and Japanese consumers. It will be interesting to see whether the rest of the world flocks as avidly as Americans do to fast food restaurants.

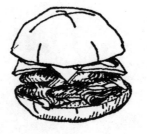

Chapter Three

FAST FOOD RESTAURANT CALORIE COUNTS

ARBY'S

Food	Calories
Beef and cheese sandwich	450
Club sandwich	560
Ham'n cheese sandwich	380
Junior roast beef sandwich	220
Roast beef sandwich	350
Super roast beef sandwich	620
Swiss king sandwich	660
Turkey deluxe sandwich	510
Turkey sandwich	410

ARTHUR TREACHER'S

Food	Calories
Chicken	271
Chicken sandwich	265
Chips	243
Chowder	66
Cole slaw	144
Fish	241
Fish sandwich	282
Krunch pup	358
Lemon luvs	324
Shrimp	331

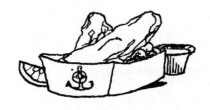

BASKIN ROBBINS

Food	Calories
One scoop with sugar cone:	
Banana dacquiri ice	129
Butter pecan	195
Chocolate fudge	229
Chocolate mint	189
Fresh peach	165
Fresh strawberry	168
Fresh vanilla	217
Jamoca	182
Mango sherbet	132
Rocky road	204

BRIDGEMAN'S

Food	Calories
Vanilla ice cream with plain cone	170
Vanilla ice cream with sugar cone	200

A Bridgeman's spokesman said "Calorie content does not increase appreciably for other flavors."

BURGER CHEF

Food	Calories
Big Chef	569
Cheeseburger	290
Double cheeseburger	420
French fries	
Large	351
Regular	250
Fish fillet	547
Hamburger	244
Mariner platter	734
Rancher platter	640
Salad	
Lettuce and carrots	18
Super Chef	563
Top Chef	661
Beverages	
Coffee (8 oz)	2
Hot cocoa (8 oz)	198

Milk
2% fat (8 oz)	112
Whole (8 oz)	138

Shakes
Chocolate (12 oz)	403
Vanilla (12 oz)	380

Condiments
Cheese
American (1 tbsp)	21
Parmesan (1 tbsp)	25
Cherry tomatoes	6
Croutons	130
Garbanzo beans	102
Green peppers	6
Raw alfalfa sprouts	11.64
Shoestring beets (2 oz)	18

BURGER KING

Food	Calories
Apple pie	240
Beef sandwich	644
Cheeseburger	350
Chicken sandwich	620
Double beef whopper	850
With cheese	950
Double cheeseburger	530
Fish sandwich	646
French fries	210
Ham and cheese sandwich	573
Hamburger	290
Milk	150
Onion rings	270
Shake	340
Whopper	630
With cheese	740
Whopper junior	370
With cheese	420

CARL'S JR

Food	Calories
American cheese slice	40
Apple turnover	330
California roast beef	380
Carrot cake	380
Chili cheese dog	400
Chili dog	360
Famous star hamburger	480
Fish fillet sandwich	550
French fries	220
Happy star hamburger	290
Old time star hamburger	440
Onion rings	320
Original hot dog	340
Salad	170
Shake	310
Steak sandwich	630
Super star hamburger	660

CHURCH'S FRIED CHICKEN

Food	Calories
Apple pie	300
Chicken snack	316
Cole slaw	83
Corn on the cob	165
Dinner roll	83
French fries	256
Jalapeno pepper	4
Pecan pie	367

DAIRY QUEEN

Food	Calories
Banana split	540
Big Brazier	
Deluxe	470
Regular	457
With cheese	553
Brazier cheese dog	330
Brazier chili dog	330
Brazier dog	273
Brazier french fries	
Large	320
Small	200
Brazier onion rings	300
Brazier regular	260
Brazier with cheese	318
Buster bar	390
Cone	
Large	340
Regular	230
Small	110

Dipped cone
- Large   450
- Regular   300
- Small   150

DQ float   330

DQ freeze   520

DQ parfait   460

DQ sandwich   140

Dilly bar   240

Fiesta sundae   570

Malt
- Large   840
- Regular   600
- Small   340

Mr. Misty
- Float   440
- Freeze   500
- Kiss   70

Sundae
- Large   400
- Regular   290
- Small   170

Super Brazier	783
Chili dog	555
Dog	518
Dog with cheese	593

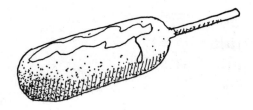

DUNKIN' DONUTS

Food	Calories
Cake and chocolate cake donuts (includes rings, sticks, crullers, etc.)	240
Fancies[1] (includes coffee rolls, danish, etc.)	215
Munchkins[2]	
Cake and chocolate cake	66
Yeast raised	26
Yeast raised donuts[3]	160

[1] Add 40-50 calories per donut for filling and topping combined.

[2] Add 10-15 calories per munchkin for filling and topping combined.

[3] Add 5-10 calories per donut for glaze.

FRIENDLY ICE CREAM

Food	Calories
Big Burger	
With cheese	480
Without cheese	420
Bounty Burger	570
Cole slaw	80
Cones	
Cake	
Regular (4 oz.)	
Chocolate	260
Vanilla	250
Double dip (7 oz.)	
Chocolate	440
Vanilla	420
Sugar	
Regular (4 oz.)	
Chocolate	310
Vanilla	290
Double dip (7 oz.)	
Chocolate	490
Vanilla	460
Fish	340

French fries	125
Fribble	
Chocolate	470
Vanilla	420
Ham and cheese	400
Hamburger	260
Sundae	
Fudge/Vanilla	420
Strawberry/Vanilla	340

GINO'S

Food	Calories
Apple pie	198
Cheese sirloiner	526
Cheese steak	496
Cheeseburger	295
Coke	
Giant	181
Regular	117
Dessert	
Cheesecake	210
Chocolate	250
Strawberry	210
Dinner roll	51
Fish platter	650
Fish sandwich	445
French fries	
Giant	274
Regular	195
Giant sirloiner	526
Hamburger	249

Home style hamburger	513
Kentucky fried chicken	290
Orange	
Giant	217
Regular	140
Roast beef	413
Root beer	
Giant	190
Regular	122
Sirloiner	436

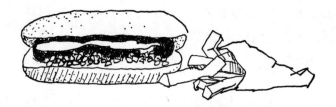

HARDEE'S

Food	Calories
Apple turnover	282
Big cheese	495
Big deluxe	546
Big fish sandwich	514
Big roast beef	418
Big twin	447
Biscuit	274.64
With egg	383
With jelly	324
Cheeseburger	335
Chicken fillet	510.15
Egg (medium)	108
French fries	
Large	381
Small	239
Ham and cheese	376.10
Ham biscuit	349.47
With egg	458
Hamburger	305

Hot dog	346
Jelly	49
Milkshake	391
Roast beef sandwich	376
Sausage biscuit	413.10
With egg	527
Steak biscuit	419.44
With egg	527

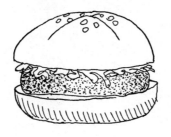

HOWARD JOHNSON'S

Food	Calories
Cone - large	
Chocolate	390
Vanilla	370
- medium	
Chocolate	261
Vanilla	247
- small	
Chocolate	195
Vanilla	186
Fried clams - 7 oz.	357
Pecan pie - one-eighth	474
Sherbet	357

JACK IN THE BOX

Food	Calories
Apple turnover	411
Breakfast jack sandwich	301
Bonus jack hamburger	461
Cheeseburger	310
Deluxe	314
Double cheese omelette	414
French fries	270
French toast breakfast	537
Ham and cheese omelette	425
Hamburger	263
Deluxe	260
Jack burrito	448
Jack steak sandwich	428
Jumbo jack hamburger	551
With cheese	628
Lemon turnover	446
Moby jack sandwich	455
Onion rings	351
Pancake breakfast	626

Ranchero style omelette	414
Scrambled egg breakfast	719
Shake	
Chocolate	325
Strawberry	323
Vanilla	317
Taco	
Regular	189
Super	285

KENTUCKY FRIED CHICKEN

Food	Calories	
	Original Recipe	Extra Crispy
Side breast	199	286
Drumstick	117	155
Keel	236	297
Rib	241.39	
Thigh	257	343
Wing	136	201
9 pieces chicken	1892.24	
Chicken dinner*	830	950

*Dinner comprises mashed potatoes and gravy, cole slaw, roll and 3 pieces of chicken either 1.) wing, rib and thigh; 2.) wing, drumstick and thigh; or 3.) wing, drumstick and keel.

LONG JOHN SILVER'S

Food	Calories
Breaded clams	617
Breaded oysters	441
Carbonated drinks (10 oz)	120
Chicken planks	457
With fries	745
Clam chowder (8 oz)	107
Clam dinner	891
Cole slaw	138
Corn on the cob	176
Diet carbonated drinks (10 oz)	less than 10
Fish and chicken dinner	837
Fish/Fryes	837
Fish/More	894
Fish sandwich	337
French Fryes	288
Fish with batter	
2 pieces	366
3 pieces	549

Hush puppies	153
Milk (8 oz)	159
Non-carbonated drinks (10 oz)	120
Ocean scallops	283
Oyster dinner	867
Peg legs with batter	350
With fries	725
Scallop dinner	709
Seafood platter	894
Shrimp with batter	268
Treasure chest	506

McDONALD'S

Food	Calories
Big Mac	563
Cheeseburger	307
Cones	
Cake	185
Sugar	170
Cookies	
Chocolaty chips	342
McDonaldland	308
Egg McMuffin	327
English muffin	187
Filet-o-fish	432
French fries	220
Hamburger	220
Hash browns	125
Hotcakes with butter/syrup	500
Pie	
Apple	253
Cherry	260
Quarter pounder	424
With cheese	524

| Sausage | 206 |
| Scrambled eggs | 180 |

Shakes
Chocolate	383
Strawberry	362
Vanilla	352

Sundaes
Caramel	328
Hot fudge	310
Strawberry	289

PIZZA HUT

Food	Calories	
	Thin/ Crispy	Thick/ Chewy
Standard		
Cheese	180	208
Pepperoni	202	224
Pork/Mushroom	196	227
Super supreme	266	300
Superstyle		
Cheese	213	235
Pepperoni	233	244
Pork/Mushroom	230	244
Supreme	216	244

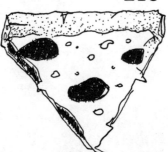

This data is computed for one slice of a medium pizza which consists of eight slices per pizza.

PONDEROSA

Food	Calories	
	Entree	Dinner
Chopped beef (chopped beef, baked potato, lettuce, tomato, onions, kaiser roll)	324	726.8
Double deluxe (steakhouse deluxe bun, french fries, dill pickles, tomato slices, lettuce)	362	791.3
Extra-cut prime rib (baked potato, lettuce, tomato, onions, kaiser roll)	408.98	811.78
Extra-cut rib eye (baked potato, lettuce, tomato, onions, kaiser roll)	358	760.8
Fillet of sole dinner (baked potato, lettuce, tomato, onions, kaiser roll)	250.8	653.6
Fillet of sole sandwich (steakhouse deluxe bun, french fries, lemon wedge)	125.4	550.8

Junior patty   98   445.9
    (Junior bun, french fries)

Prime rib   286   688.8
    (baked potato, lettuce, tomato, onions, kaiser roll)

Rib eye   259   661.8
    (baked potato, lettuce, tomato, onions, kaiser roll)

Rib eye/Shrimp   259-139   800.8
    (baked potato, lettuce, tomato, onions, kaiser roll)

Shrimp   220   622.8
    (baked potato, lettuce, tomato, onions, kaiser roll)

Steakhouse deluxe   181   610.8
    (steakhouse deluxe bun, french fries, dill pickles, tomato slices, lettuce)

Strip sirloin   277   679.8
    (baked potato, lettuce, tomato, onions, kaiser roll)

Super sirloin   383   785.8
    (baked potato, lettuce, tomato, onions, kaiser roll)

T-bone	374	776.8

(baked potato, lettuce, tomato, onions, kaiser roll)

Beverages	Calories
Coca-Cola - 8 oz.	96
Coffee	2
Dr. Pepper - 8 oz.	96
Milk - 8 oz.	159
Rootbeer - 8 oz.	104
Sprite - 8 oz.	95
Tea	2

Miscellaneous

Baked potato	145
Butter	36
Catsup - 1 T.	18
Cocktail sauce - ½ oz.	57
Dill pickles - 3	1.5
French fries	230.4
Kaiser roll	184
Lemon wedge	5

Lettuce - 0.5 oz.	1.5
- 3.0 oz.	11.8
Margarine - 1 T.	36
Mayonnaise - 1 T.	101
Mustard	4
Onion	4
Salad dressing	
Blue cheese - 7/16 oz.	56
Creamy Italian - 7/16 oz.	60
French - 7/16 oz.	56
Oil and vinegar - 7/16 oz.	54
Thousand Island	
- 7/16 oz.	51
Steak sauce - 7/16 oz.	10
Steakhouse deluxe bun	190
Tartar sauce - 1 T.	95
Tomato - small	22
- two slices	5.5
Worcestershire sauce	4

POPPIN' FRESH

Food	Calories
Chef's salad	800
Custard pie - one-sixth	380
Dairy salad	650
Dinner salad	250
Doughboy salad	530
Pumpkin pie - one-sixth	390
Shrimp salad	640
Tuna salad	640

RED BARN

Food	Calories
Apple pie	217
Cheese buster	707
French fries	108
Salad	189
Shake	358

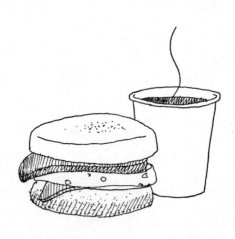

RED LOBSTER

Food	Calories
Albacore tuna	107-185
Breaded fried pollock or whiting	175-200
Catfish, fresh-water	78-117
Chicken, fried - 4 pieces	452
Clams	89
Cod	79-97
Crab, Snow	93
Egg	163
Flounder	84-90
Garlic bread - 1 slice	136
Grouper	83-94
Haddock	79
Halibut	77
Hamburger pattie	268
Hush puppies - 2	206
Lobster	95
Oysters	54-92

Perch	88
Polloch	86-94
Potato	76
Scallops	87
Shrimp	88-97
Sirloin steak	353
Snapper	100-105
Sole	80-85
Tuna, other	122-126
Turbot	94
Whiting	105

Broiled fisherman's platter   992
    (lobster, sea bass, scallops, deviled
    crab, hush puppies, cole slaw and
    baked potato)

Broiled stuffed flounder   1027.8
    (fillets stuffed with crab meat filling,
    hush puppies, cole slaw and baked
    potato)

Mariner's platter   944.3
    (fried shrimp, fish fillet, oysters, fish
    fingers, deviled crab cake, fried fish

fillet, hush puppies, cole slaw and
baked potato)

Sampler platter   808.3
(broiled lobster, broiled Alaskan
split crab legs, fried shrimp, hush
puppies, cole slaw and baked potato)

Shore platter   832.5
(fried shrimp, scallops, oysters, fish
fillet, hush puppies, cole slaw and
baked potato)

Steak and lobster   1539.8
(sirloin steak, broiled rock lobster
tail, hush puppies, cole slaw and
baked potato)

RUSTLER STEAK HOUSE

Food	Calories
Baked potato	231
Dressing	
Blue cheese	151
French	122
Italian	166
Thousand Island	150
Jello	
Cherry	75
Pickle	2
Potato chips	82
Pudding	
Chocolate	144
Roll with butter	40
Rustler	120
Twisted	182
Rib eye	369

SHAKEY'S

Pizza	Calories
1 serving is 1/10 of a 13-inch pizza.	
Anchovy	151
Bacon and pineapple	172
Bacon, mushroom and tomato	172
Beef and onion	164
Black olive	162
Canadian bacon	168
Cheese	154
Chorizo and green pepper	166
Chorizo and jalapeno	167
Combination	185
With anchovy	191
Green peppers and pimento	144
Italian salami	173
Italian sausage	167
With mushrooms	169
With olives	178
Louisiana shrimp	148
Mushroom	143
With olives and shrimp	156

STEAK N SHAKE

Food	Calories
Baked beans	173
Baked ham sandwich	450
Chili	336
Chili Mac	310
Chili Three Ways	401
Cottage cheese	93
Egg sandwich	274
French fries	211
Ham and egg sandwich	434
Ketchup	12
Lettuce	2
Lettuce and tomato salad	
With dressing	168
Low calorie platter	292
Oyster crackers	87
Saltine crackers - 3 squares	50
Steakburger	
With cheese	352
Without cheese	276

Super steakburger
  With cheese   457
  Without cheese   375
Toasted cheese sandwich   249
Triple steakburger
  With cheese   628
  Without cheese   474

Miscellaneous

Apple danish   391
Apple pie   407
Brownie   258
Brownie fudge sundae   645
Cheese cake   368
Cheese cake
  with strawberries   386
Cherry pie   334
Cherry pie ala mode   476
Chocolate shake   608
Hot fudge nut sundae   530
Ice cream   213
Lemon drink   86
Lemon float   555

Lemon freeze	548
Orange drink	83
Orange float	502
Orange freeze	516
Strawberry shake	648
Strawberry sundae	320
Vanilla ice cream	213
Vanilla shake	619

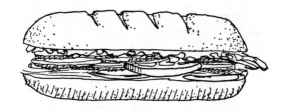

TACO BELL

Food	Calories
Bean burrito	343
Beef burrito	466
Beefy tostada	291
Bellbeefer	221
Bellbeefer - with cheese	278
Burrito supreme	457
Combination burrito	404
Enchirito	454
Pintos 'n cheese	168
Taco	186
Tostada	179

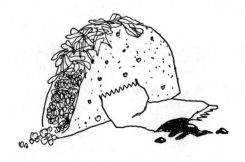

TACO CHARLEY

Food	Calories
Bean burrito	
Mild	360
Spicy	370
Beef burrito	
Mild	430
Spicy	430
Burrito grande	460
Charley	280
Combination burrito	
Mild	415
Spicy	420
Crisp taco	200
Enchilada	350
Friyoles	250
Soft taco	200
Tortilla chips	170
Tosta grande	300
Tostada	200

TACO JOHN'S

Food	Calories
Taco	184
Softshell	305
Regular burrito	337
Beefy burrito	447
Combination burrito	417
Taco burger	315
Taco bravo	403
Enchilada	358
Tostada	212
Beefy tostada	315
Combination tostada	263
Chili & fritos	330
Texas chili	247
Refried beans	313
Taco salad	138
Taco salad w/meat	236
Apple grande	280
Super burrito	246
"As a Dinner"	246

WENDYS

Food	Calories
Cheeseburger	
Single cheese	580
Double cheese	800
Triple cheese	1040
Chili	230
French fries	330
Frosty	390
Hamburger	
Single	470
Double	670
Triple	850

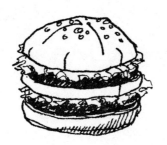

WHITE CASTLE

Food	Calories
Bun	65.03
Cheeseburger	185.34
Fish - without tartar sauce	192.03
French fries	225.47
Hamburger	160.01

WIENERSCHNITZEL

Food	Calories
Chili cheese dog	311
Chili dog	269
Corn dog	520
French fries	215
Hot apple pie	350
Kraut dog	241
Polish sandwich	404
Super deluxe	472

ZANTIGO

Food	Calories
Burrito	345
Enchirito	391
Frijoles	231
Taco	146
Tostada	206

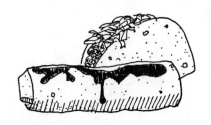

SECTION

TWO

DIABETIC FOOD EXCHANGE VALUES

Control of food consumption is the most essential and often the most difficult part of treating diabetes.

Because diabetes is a chronic, incurable disease, diet control for the patient must be continuous. The aim in treating this disease is to establish normal blood sugar levels, which is impossible unless food intake is regulated.

Diabetics must follow a diet that avoids meals with concentrated carbohydrates (sugars and starches) and other foods containing excessive calories. In the following pages, dietary information for fast food restaurants is provided for diabetics. The information is given in terms of food exchanges. For example, in the first chart a club sandwich is cited as having 3 bread food exchange values. Since one bread exchange (one slice of bread or one small baked potato) has 15 grams of carbohydrates, the club sandwich's three bread values would equal 45 grams of carbohydrates. Similarly, one meat exchange is one ounce of meat. The club sandwich's three meat values would equal three ounces of meat.

Because of the high values cited in the following pages, diabetics must be even more careful than the average consumer in not overeating when partaking of high calorie meals in fast food restaurants.

ARBY'S	Bread	Fat	Meat
Beef and Cheese Sandwich	1½		1½
Club Sandwich	3	3	3
Ham 'n Cheese Sandwich	2		2½
Junior Roast Beef Sandwich	1½		1½
Roast Beef Sandwich	2		2½
Super Roast Beef Sandwich	4	2	3
Swiss King Sandwich	3½	2½	4
Turkey Deluxe Sandwich	3	3	3*
Turkey Sandwich	2½	2	3*

*Meat exchange is lean meat, while all other exchanges are medium fat meat.

BURGER CHEF	Bread	Fat	Meat
Big Chef	2	3	3
Cheeseburger	1½	1	2
Double Cheeseburger	1½	2	3
French Fries	1½	2	
Hamburger	1½		2

BURGER KING	Bread	Fat	Meat
Cheeseburger	1½	1	2
French Fries - small	2	2	
Hamburger	1½		2
Hot dog	1½	2	1*
Whopper	3	4	3

*High fat meat exchange rather than medium fat meat exchange.

DAIRY QUEEN	Bread	Fat	Meat
Big Brazier regular	2½	1	3
Big Brazier w/Cheese	2½	1	4
Brazier Dog w/Cheese	1½	1	2
Brazier Dog w/Chili	1½	1	2
Brazier French Fries			
small	1½	2	
large	3	3	
Brazier Onion Rings	2	3	
DQ Choc. Dipped Cone			
small	1½	1	
DQ Choc. Malt - small	3½	2	
DQ Choc. Sundae			
small	2	1	
medium	3½	1	
DQ Cone			
small	1	1	
medium	2½	1½	
large	3½	2	
DQ Sandwich	1½	1	
Dilly Bar	1½	3	
Fish Sandwich	3	1	2
Super Brazier	2½	2	6
Brazier Dog	1½	1½	1

KENTUCKY FRIED CHICKEN	Bread	Fat	Meat
Drumstick - original recipe			2
Keel - original recipe			3
Rib - original recipe	½		2½
Thigh - original recipe	1		3
Wing - original recipe		1	1½
Chicken Dinner			
original recipe	4	3	6
extra crispy	4	5	6

LONG JOHN SILVER'S	Bread	Fat	Meat
Breaded Clams	3	4	1
Breaded Oysters	4	2	1
Chicken Planks	2	2	3
Cole Slaw	1	1	
Fish - w/Batter (2)	1	2	2
w/Batter (3)	2	2	3
Shrimp - w/Batter (6)	2	1	1

MCDONALD'S	Bread	Fat	Meat
Apple pie	2	4	
Big Mac	2½	3	3
Cheeseburger	2		2
Chocolate Shake	4	2	
Egg McMuffin	1½	2	2
English Muffin - buttered	2		1
Fillet 'O Fish	2	3	1½
French Fries	1½		2
Hamburger	2		1½
Quarter Pounder	2	1	3
Quarter Pounder w/Cheese	2	2	4
Sausage - pork		2	1*
Scrambled Eggs			2

*High fat meat exchange rather than medium fat meat exchange.

PIZZA HUT	Bread	Fat	Meat
Thin and Crispy			
Standard			
Cheese	1½		1
Pepperoni	1		1
(½ vegetable ½ fruit)*			
Pork/Mushroom	1		1
(½ vegetable)			
Super Supreme	1		1½
(1 vegetable ½ fruit)			
Superstyle			
Cheese	1	½	1½
(1 fruit)			
Pepperoni	1	½	1
(1½ vegetable)			
Pork/Mushroom	1½	½	1½
Supreme	1	½	1
(1 vegetable ½ fruit)			
Thick and Chewy			
Standard			
Cheese	1½		1
(1 vegetable)			
Pepperoni	1		1½
(1 fruit)			
Pork/Mushroom	1½	½	1½
(1 fruit)			

*Other forms of food exchanges not listed as a separate heading at the top of the page.

PIZZA HUT CON'T.	Bread	Fat	Meat
Thick and Chewy			
Super Supreme	1½	½	2
(½ fruit)			
Superstyle			
Cheese	1½	½	1½
(1 vegetable)			
Pepperoni	1	1	1½
(1 vegetable ½ fruit)			
Pork/Mushroom	1	1	1½
(1 vegetable ½ fruit)			
Supreme	1	1	1½
(1 vegetable ½ fruit)			

POPPIN' FRESH	Bread	Fat	Meat
Chef's Salad	2	5	6
Custard Pie (1/6)	3	4	
Dairy Salad	2	2	5
Dinner Salad	1	4	
Doughboy Salad	2	7	1
Pumpkin Pie (1/6)	4	3	
Shrimp Salad	1	7	3
(1 vegetable)*			
Tuna Salad	2	5	3
(1 vegetable)			

*Another food exchange value heading not listed as a heading at the top of the page.

87

STEAK N SHAKE	Bread	Fat	Meat
Baked Beans	2		1
Baked Ham Sandwich	2½	1	3
Chili	2½	1	2
Chili Mac	2		2
Chili Three Ways	3	2	2
Cottage Cheese		(-1)	2
Egg Sandwich	2	1	1
French Fries	2		2
Ham and Egg Sandwich	2		4
Ketchup			
(1/3 fruit)*			
Lettuce and Tomato Salad			
w/Dressing		3	
(½ fruit)			
Low Calorie Platter			5
Mayonnaise		2½	
Oyster Crackers	1		
Saltine Crackers	½		
Steakburger	2		2
w/Cheese	2		3
Super Steakburger	2	(-1)	4
w/Cheese	2	(-1)	5

*Another food exchange heading not listed at the top of the page.

88

STEAK N SHAKE CON'T.

	Bread	Fat	Meat
1000 Island Dressing		6	
(1 fruit)			
Toasted Cheese Sandwich	1½	2	1
Triple Steakburger	2		5
w/Cheese	2		7

Miscellaneous

	Bread	Fat	Meat
Apple Danish	2½	5	
Apple Pie	2½	3	
(2 fruit)			
Brownie	2½	2	
Brownie Fudge Sundae	4½	7	
Cheese Cake	4	2	
Cheese Cake			
w/Strawberries	3½	2	
(1 fruit)			
Cherry Pie	2½	3	
(1 fruit)			
Cherry Pie ala Mode	3½	4	
(1 fruit)			
Chocolate Shake	3	5½	
(1 milk)			
Hot Fudge Nut Sundae	3	6	
(½ milk)			

STEAK N SHAKE CON'T.	Bread	Fat	Meat
Ice Cream	1½	2½	
Lemon Drink (2 fruit)			
Lemon Float (1 fruit 1 milk)	4	1½	
Lemon Freeze (1 fruit 1 milk)	2½	3	
Orange Drink (1 fruit)			
Orange Float (1 fruit 1 milk)	3½	1	
Orange Freeze (1 fruit 1 milk)	2½	3	
Strawberry Shake (1 fruit 1 milk)	2½	6	
Strawberry Sundae (1 fruit)	1½	5	
Vanilla Shake (1 milk)	3	5½	

*Another food exchange heading not listed at the top of the page.

TACO BELL	Bread	Fat	Meat
Bean Burrito	3	2	1
Beef Burrito	2½	1	3
Beefy Tostada	1½	1	2
Burrito Supreme	3	2	2
Combination Burrito	3	1	2
Pintos 'N Cheese	1½		1
Taco	1		1½
Tostada	1½		1

WENDY'S	Bread	Fat	Meat
Cheeseburger			
Single	2	2	4
Triple	2	2	10
Chili	1½		3*
French Fries	3	3	
Hamburger			
Single	2	2	3
Double	2	1	6
Triple	2		9

*Lean meat exchange rather than medium fat meat exchange like the other items listed.

WHITE CASTLE	Bread	Fat	Meat
Cheeseburger	1		1*
Fish without tartar sauce	1½	1	½
French Fries	2	2	
Hamburger	1	1	½

*High fat meat exchange rather than lean meat exchange like the other two listed items.

SECTION

THREE

NUTRITIONAL ANALYSIS
OF FAST FOODS

ARBY'S

	Protein (g)	Carbohydrates (g)	Fat (g)	Sodium (mg)	Cholesterol (mg)
Beef and Cheese	27	36	22	1220	55
Club Sandwich	30	43	30	1610	100
Ham 'n Cheese	23	33	17	1350	60
Junior Roast Beef Sandwich	12	21	9	530	35
Roast Beef Sandwich	22	32	15	880	45
Super Roast Beef	30	61	28	1420	85
Swiss King Sandwich	34	55	34	1585	100
Turkey Deluxe	28	46	24	1220	70
Turkey Sandwich	24	36	19	1060	70

ARTHUR TREACHER'S

	Protein (g)	Carbohydrates (g)	Fat (g)	Sodium (mg)	Cholesterol (mg)
Chicken	19.9	12.1	15.9	240	47.4
Chicken Sandwich	10.4	28.2	12.3	454	20.5
Chips	3.5	30.8	11.6	347	0.6
Chowder	2.7	6.6	3.2	491	5.3
Cole Slaw	1.2	13.1	9.6	312	7.7
Fish	13.0	17.2	13.4	305	37.8
Fish Sandwich	10.5	25.3	15.4	491	5.3
Krunch Pup	9.5	21.2	26.1	786	44.1
Lemon Luvs	3.1	41.2	16.3	369	0.5
Shrimp	11.4	23.6	21.2	467	80.7

BURGER CHEF

	Hamburger	Cheeseburger	Double Cheese	Big Chef	Super Chef
Protein (g)	11.5	14.4	24.3	23.2	29.3
Carbohydrate (g)	29.1	29.3	29.5	38.1	44.3
Fat (g)	8.9	12.6	22.3	35.9	29.6
Vitamin A (IU)	114	267	431	279	754
Vitamin B_1 (mg)	.16	.21	.32	.31	.40
Vitamin B_2 (mg)	.17	.17	.20	.26	.30
Niacin (mg)	2.8	2.8	4.4	4.7	6.0
Vitamin B_6 (mg)	.16	.17	.31	36.7	.45
Vitamin B_{12} (mg)	.26	.36	.72	.62	.87
Folacin (mg)	21.1	23.3	26.7	36.7	52.4
Panthothenic (mg)	.28	.33	.51	.54	.79
Vitamin C (mg)	1.2	1.2	1.2	1.0	9.3
Vitamin D (mg)	-	-	-	-	-
Vitamin E (mg)	-	-	-	-	-
Calcium (mg)	45	132	222	152	205
Iodine (mg)	-	-	-	-	-
Iron (mg)	2	2.2	3.2	3.6	4.4
Potassium (mg)	209	219	360	382	578
Magnesium (mg)	8.9	8.9	15	13.6	25.4
Sodium (mg)	394	536	692	718	793
Cholesterol (mg)	27.4	38.7	77.4	80.6	104

BURGER CHEF CONTINUED

	Top Chef	Reg. Fries	Large Fries	Fish fillet	Mariner Platter
Protein (g)	40.5	2.4	3.4	21.3	29
Carbohydrate (g)	36.4	19.9	27.8	45.6	78.3
Fat (g)	38.1	18.6	26	30.8	34
Vitamin A (IU)	273	0	0	400	2070.0
Vitamin B_1 (mg)	.47	.04	.06	.22	.23
Vitamin B_2 (mg)	.35	.07	.10	.23	.34
Niacin (mg)	8.1	1.7	2.4	2.7	5.2
Vitamin B_6 (mg)	.56	-	-	.04	.09
Vitamin B_{12} (mg)	1.16	-	-	.10	.56
Folacin (mg)	34	13.4	18.8	31.9	63.9
Panthothenic (mg)	.78	0	0	.23	.26
Vitamin C (mg)	-	11.5	16.2	1.0	23.5
Vitamin D (mg)	-	-	-	-	-
Vitamin E (mg)	-	-	-	-	-
Calcium (mg)	194	9	13	145	63
Iodine (mg)	-	-	-	-	-
Iron (mg)	5.4	.7	.9	2.2	3.3
Potassium (mg)	612	473	661	271	996
Magnesium (mg)	26.4	15.6	21.8	19	49
Sodium (mg)	722	242	338	595	336
Cholesterol (mg)	134	-	-	43.2	35

98

BURGER CHEF CONTINUED

	Rancher Platter	Salad
Protein (g)	32.4	1.0
Carbohydrate (g)	33.1	4.1
Fat (g)	42.2	.1
Vitamin A (IU)	1751.0	1702.0
Vitamin B$_1$ (mg)	.38	.06
Vitamin B$_2$ (mg)	.29	.07
Niacin (mg)	8.6	.4
Vitamin B$_6$ (mg)	.61	.07
Vitamin B$_{12}$ (mg)	1.01	0
Folacin (mg)	68	40.7
Panthothenic (mg)	.82	.23
Vitamin C (mg)	23.5	6.9
Vitamin D (mg)	0	0
Vitamin E (mg)	0	0
Calcium (mg)	66	24
Iodine (mg)	0	0
Iron (mg)	5.3	.6
Potassium (mg)	1238.0	216
Magnesium (mg)	53	13.7
Sodium (mg)	396	15
Cholesterol (mg)	105	0

BURGER KING

	Cheeseburger	French Fries	Hamburger	Hot Dog
Protein (g)	17	3	14	11
Carbohydrate (g)	29	28	29	23
Fat (g)	13	10	9	17
Vitamin A (IU)	195		21	
Vitamin B$_1$ (mg)				
Vitamin B$_2$ (mg)				
Niacin (mg)	2.2	2.4	2.2	2
Vitamin C (mg)	0.5	16	0.5	
Calcium (mg)	141	12	45	40
Iron (mg)	2	1	2	2
Potassium (mg)	219	666	208	170
Phosphorus (mg)	229	87	119	117
Sodium (mg)	562	5	401	841

BURGER KING CON'T.

	Vanilla Shake	Whaler	Whopper
Protein (g)	11	18	29
Carbohydrate (g)	50	64	51
Fat (g)	11	46	32
Vitamin A (IU)	9	141	641
Vitamin B$_1$ (mg)			
Vitamin B$_2$ (mg)	0.1		
Niacin (mg)	0.3	1	5.2
Vitamin C (mg)		1.3	16
Calcium (mg)	390	70	37
Iron (mg)	0.2	1	6
Potassium (mg)	520	130	653
Phosphorus (mg)	303	91	205
Sodium (mg)	159	735	909

DAIRY QUEEN

	Banana Split	Big Brazier Deluxe	Big Brazier Regular	Big Brazier w/Cheese
Protein (g)	10	28	27	32
Carbohydrate (g)	91	36	37	38
Fat (g)	15	24	23	30
Vitamin A (IU)	750			495
Vitamin B$_1$ (mg)	0.6	0.3	0.4	0.3
Vitamin B$_2$ (mg)	0.6	0.4	0.4	0.5
Niacin (mg)	0.8	9.6	9.6	9.5
Vitamin B$_6$ (mg)	0.5	0.4	0.3	0.4
Vitamin B$_{12}$ (mg)	0.9	2.6	2.3	2.9
Vitamin C (mg)	18	2.5	2	2.3
Vitamin D (mg)		30	31	36
Calcium (mg)	350	111	113	268
Copper (mg)	0.2	0.2	0.2	0.2
Iron (mg)	1.8	5.2	5.2	5.2
Magnesium (mg)	60	45	42	47
Phosphorus (mg)	250	262	223	359
Sodium (mg)		920	910	1435
Zinc (mg)	2.3	5.5	5.4	5.9

DAIRY QUEEN CON'T.

	Brazier with Cheese	Brazier Cheese Dog	Brazier Chili Dog	Brazier Dog
Protein (g)	18	15	13	11
Carbohydrate (g)	30	24	25	23
Fat (mg)	14	19	20	15
Vitamin A (IU)				
Vitamin B_1 (mg)	0.3		0.2	0.1
Vitamin B_2 (mg)	0.3	0.2	0.2	0.2
Niacin (mg)	5.7	3.3	3.9	2.6
Vitamin B_6 (mg)	0.1	0.1	0.2	0.1
Vitamin B_{12} (mg)	1.2	1.2	1.3	1.1
Vitamin C (mg)	1.2		11	11
Vitamin D (mg)	13	23	20	23
Calcium (mg)	163	168	86	75
Copper (mg)	0.1	0.1	0.1	0.8
Iron (mg)	3.5	1.6	2	1.5
Magnesium (mg)	26	24	38	21
Phosphorus (mg)	192	182	139	104
Sodium (mg)	865		939	868
Zinc (mg)	2.8	1.9	1.8	1.4

DAIRY QUEEN CON'T.

	B. French Fries (sm)	B. French Fries (lg)	B. Onion Rings	B. Regular
Protein (g)	2	3	6	13
Carbohydrate (g)	25	40	33	28
Fat (g)	10	16	17	9
Vitamin A (IU)				
Vitamin B_1 (mg)	0.1	0.1	0.1	0.3
Vitamin B_2 (mg)				0.3
Niacin (mg)	0.8	1.2	0.4	5
Vitamin B_6 (mg)	0.2	0.3	0.1	0.1
Vitamin B_{12} (mg)				1
Vitamin C (mg)	3.6	4.8	2.4	1
Vitamin D (mg)	16	24	8	13
Calcium (mg)			20	70
Copper (mg)		0.1	0.1	0.1
Iron (mg)	0.4	0.4	0.4	3.5
Magnesium (mg)	16	24	16	23
Phosphorus (mg)	100	150	60	114
Sodium (mg)				576
Zinc (mg)		0.3	0.3	2.3

DAIRY QUEEN CON'T.

	Buster Bar	DQ Choc. Dipped Cone (sm)	DQ Choc. Dipped Cone (med)	DQ Choc. Dipped Cone (lg)
Protein (g)	10	3	7	10
Carbohydrate (g)	37	20	40	58
Fat (g)	22	7	13	20
Vitamin A (IU)	300	100	300	400
Vitamin B_1 (mg)	0.1		0.1	0.1
Vitamin B_2 (mg)	0.3	0.2	0.3	0.5
Niacin (mg)	1.6			
Vitamin B_6 (mg)	0.1		0.1	0.1
Vitamin B_{12} (mg)	0.9	0.4	0.6	0.9
Vitamin C (mg)				
Vitamin D (mg)				8
Calcium (mg)	200	100	200	300
Copper (mg)	0.2		0.1	0.1
Iron	0.7		0.4	0.4
Magnesium (mg)	60	16	24	40
Phosphorus (mg)	150	80	150	200
Sodium (mg)				
Zinc (mg)	1.2	0.3	0.6	0.9

DAIRY QUEEN CON'T.

	DQ Choc. Malt (sm)	DQ Choc. Malt (med)	DQ Choc. Malt (lg)	DQ Choc. Sundae (sm)
Protein (g)	10	15	22	4
Carbohydrate (g)	51	89	125	30
Fat (g)	11	20	28	4
Vitamin A (IU)	400	750	750	100
Vitamin B$_1$ (mg)	0.1	0.1	0.2	
Vitamin B$_2$ (mg)	0.3	0.6	0.9	0.2
Niacin (mg)	0.4	0.8	1.2	
Vitamin B$_6$ (mg)	0.2	0.2	0.3	
Vitamin B$_{12}$ (mg)	1.2	1.8	2.4	0.5
Vitamin C (mg)	2.4	3.6	6	
Vitamin D (mg)	60	100	140	
Calcium (mg)	300	500	600	100
Copper (mg)	0.1	0.1	0.2	0.1
Iron (mg)	1.8	3.6	5.4	0.7
Magnesium (mg)	40	60	80	24
Phosphorus (mg)	200	400	600	100
Sodium (mg)			.	
Zinc (mg)	1.5	3	3.8	0.6

DAIRY QUEEN CON'T.

	DQ Choc. Sundae (med)	DQ Choc. Sundae (lg)	DQ Cone (sm)	DQ Cone (med)
Protein (g)	6	9	3	6
Carbohydrate (g)	53	71	18	35
Fat (g)	7	9	3	7
Vitamin A (IU)	300	400	100	300
Vitamin B$_1$ (mg)	0.1	0.1		0.1
Vitamin B$_2$ (mg)	0.3	0.4	0.1	0.3
Niacin (mg)		0.4		
Vitamin B$_6$ (mg)	0.1	0.1		0.1
Vitamin B$_{12}$ (mg)	6	1.2	0.4	0.6
Vitamin C (mg)				
Vitamin D (mg)		8		
Calcium (mg)	200	300	100	200
Copper (mg)	0.1	0.2	0.1	0.1
Iron (mg)	3.6	5.4	0.7	1.1
Magnesium (mg)	60	80	24	32
Phosphorus (mg)	400	600	100	150
Sodium (mg)				
Zinc (mg)	3	3.8	0.6	0.9

DAIRY QUEEN CON'T.

	DQ Cone (lg)	DQ Float	DQ Freeze	DQ Parfait
Protein (g)	10	6	11	10
Carbohydrate (g)	52	59	89	81
Fat (g)	10	8	13	11
Vitamin A (IU)	400	100	200	400
Vitamin B$_1$ (mg)	0.2	0.1	0.2	0.1
Vitamin B$_2$ (mg)	0.4	0.2	0.3	0.4
Niacin (mg)				0.4
Vitamin B$_6$ (mg)	0.1			0.2
Vitamin B$_{12}$ (mg)	1.2	0.6	1.2	1.2
Vitamin C (mg)				
Vitamin D (mg)	8			8
Calcium (mg)	300	200	300	300
Copper (mg)	0.1			0.2
Iron (mg)				1.8
Magnesium (mg)	32			40
Phosphorus (mg)	200	200	250	250
Sodium (mg)				
Zinc (mg)	0.9			1.2

DAIRY QUEEN CON'T.

	DQ Sandwich	Dilly Bar	Fiesta Sundae	Fish Sandwich
Protein (g)	3	4	9	20
Carbohydrate (g)	24	22	84	41
Fat (g)	4	15	22	17
Vitamin A (IU)	100	100	200	
Vitamin B_1 (mg)		0.1	0.2	0.2
Vitamin B_2 (mg)	0.1	0.2	0.3	0.3
Niacin (mg)	0.4			3
Vitamin B_6 (mg)				0.2
Vitamin B_{12} (mg)	0.2	0.5	0.9	1.2
Vitamin C (mg)				
Vitamin D (mg)				40
Calcium (mg)	60	100	200	60
Copper (mg)		0.1		0.1
Iron (mg)	0.4	0.4		1.1
Magnesium (mg)	8	16		24
Phosphorus (mg)	60	100	200	200
Sodium (mg)				
Zinc (mg)	0.3	0.3		0.3

DAIRY QUEEN CON'T.

	Fish Sandwich w/Cheese	Hot Fudge Brownie Delight	Mr. Misty Float	Mr. Misty Freeze
Protein (g)	24	11	6	10
Carbohydrate (g)	39	83	85	87
Fat (g)	21	22	8	12
Vitamin A (IU)	100	500	120	200
Vitamin B$_1$ (mg)	0.2	0.5	0.1	0.2
Vitamin B$_2$ (mg)	0.3	0.4	0.1	0.2
Niacin (mg)	3	0.8		
Vitamin B$_6$ (mg)	0.2	0.2		
Vitamin B$_{12}$ (mg)	1.5	0.9	0.6	1.2
Vitamin C (mg)				
Vitamin D (mg)	40			
Calcium (mg)	150	300	200	300
Copper (mg)	0.1	0.2		
Iron (mg)	0.4	1.1		
Magnesium (mg)	24	40		
Phosphorus (mg)	250	250	200	200
Sodium (mg)				
Zinc (mg)	0.3	1.5		

DAIRY QUEEN CON'T.

	Super Brazier	Super B. Chili Dog	Super B. Dog	Super B. Dog w/Cheese
Protein (g)	53	23	20	26
Carbohydrate (g)	35	42	41	43
Fat (g)	48	33	30	36
Vitamin A (IU)				
Vitamin B$_1$ (mg)	0.4	0.4	0.4	0.4
Vitamin B$_2$ (mg)	0.7	0.5	0.4	0.5
Niacin (mg)	15.6	8.8	7	8.1
Vitamin B$_6$ (mg)	0.7	0.3	0.2	0.2
Vitamin B$_{12}$ (mg)	5	2.7	2.1	2.3
Vitamin C (mg)	3.2	18	14	14
Vitamin D (mg)	65	32	44	44
Calcium (mg)	282	158	158	297
Copper (mg)	0.3	0.2	0.2	0.2
Niacin (mg)	7.3	4	4.3	4.4
Magnesium (mg)	61	48	37	42
Phosphorus (mg)	518	231	195	312
Sodium (mg)	1619	1640	1552	1986
Zinc (mg)	10.5	2.8	2.8	3.5

HARDEE'S

	Hamburger	Cheeseburger	Big Deluxe	1/4 lb. Cheeseburger	Roast Beef
Protein (g)	16.50	17.17	28.90	27.98	20.48
Carbohydrates (g)	29.37	28.65	48.34	41.32	36.09
Fat (g)	13.42	16.82	26.34	40.99	16.70
Vitamin A (IU)	57	749	397	508	541
Vitamin B$_1$ (mg)	.58	.32	.73	.60	.19
Vitamin B$_2$ (mg)	.55	.51	.50	.35	.929
Niacin (mg)	6.38	5.45	10.61	14.04	3.71
Vitamin C (mg)	2	2	42.36	33.02	3.21
Calcium (mg)	23	48	98.10	102.62	56.47
Iron (mg)	3.63	2.67	6.68	6.94	6.30
Potassium (mg)	231	197	594	887	205
Sodium (mg)	682	789	1083	1950	1030
Cholesterol (mg)	0	0	77	61	57

HARDEE'S CONTINUED

	Big Roast Beef	Hot Dog	Ham & Cheese	Big Fish	Chicken Fillet
Protein (g)	27.68	11.16	376	19.63	26.87
Carbohydrates (g)	33.63	25.80	36.99	49.45	41.67
Fat (g)	19.20	21.96	15.21	26.40	26.22
Vitamin A (IU)	647	0	178	1152	1098
Vitamin B$_1$ (mg)	.22	.22	.743	1.51	.629
Vitamin B$_2$ (mg)	1.03	.29	.366	0	0
Niacin (mg)	5.22	4.20	2.531	7.24	9.45
Vitamin C (mg)	7.55	0	.086	4.91	13.17
Calcium (mg)	73.56	43.20	206	87.81	82.90
Iron (mg)	8.05	2.52	3.803	5.14	4.81
Potassium (mg)	470	120	317	290	334
Sodium (mg)	1770	744	1067	314	360
Cholesterol (mg)	60	42	59	41	57

HARDEE'S CONTINUED

	Biscuit	Sausage Biscuit	Sausage Biscuit & Egg	Steak Biscuit	Steak Biscuit & Egg
Protein (g)	4.76	10.14	16.34	13.63	19.83
Carbohydrates (g)	34.74	33.98	34.38	40.55	40.95
Fat (g)	12.96	26.29	34.89	22.52	31.12
Vitamin A (IU)	44	45	755	62	772
Vitamin B$_1$ (mg)	.238	.220	.370	.426	.576
Vitamin B$_2$ (mg)	.344	.358	.408	.339	.389
Niacin (mg)	.723	2.819	2.919	3.252	3.352
Vitamin C (mg)	.033	.0714	.071	.088	.088
Calcium (mg)	149	138	169	120	151
Iron (mg)	2.44	2.75	3.95	4.60	5.80
Potassium (mg)	116	217	287	265	335
Sodium (mg)	650	864	1033	803	973
Cholesterol (mg)	3	29	293	34	298

HARDEE'S CONTINUED

	Ham Biscuit	Ham Biscuit & Egg	One Fried Egg
Protein (g)	12.36	18.56	6.20
Carbohydrates (g)	36.96	37.36	.40
Fat (g)	16.91	25.51	8.60
Vitamin A (IU)	127	837	710
Vitamin B$_1$ (mg)	.423	.573	.15
Vitamin B$_2$ (mg)	.600	.650	.05
Niacin (mg)	1.811	1.911	.10
Vitamin C (mg)	.056	.056	0
Calcium (mg)	181	211	30
Iron (mg)	3.16	4.36	1.20
Potassium (mg)	235	305	70
Sodium (mg)	1414	1584	169
Cholesterol (mg)	29	293	264

FRIENDLY ICE CREAM

	Protein (g)	Carbohydrate (g)	Fat (g)
Big Burger	36	33	15
Big Burger w/Cheese	40	34	19
Bounty Burger	37	40	28
Cole Slaw	1	6	7
Cake Cone Chocolate (sm)	5	32	13
Cake Cone Vanilla (sm) .	4	29	13
Cake Cone Double Chocolate	8	54	23
Cake Cone Double Vanilla	7	49	22
Sugar Cone Chocolate	5	41	14
Sugar Cone Vanilla	4	38	14
Sugar Cone Double Chocolate	8	63	24
Sugar Cone Double Vanilla	7	57	23
Fish	14	31	17
French Fries	20	16	6
Fribble Chocolate	11	86	10
Fribble Vanilla	10	73	10
Ham and Cheese	20	26	24
Hamburger	18	29	7
Sundae Fudge/Vanilla	7	50	22
Sundae Strawberry/Vanilla	5	39	18

KENTUCKY FRIED CHICKEN

	Wing	Drumstick	Side Breast	Thigh
Protein (g)	9.6	12.1	16.2	18.4
Carbohydrates (g)	4.2	2.6	7.1	6.5
Fat (g)	9.0	6.5	11.7	17.5
Vitamin A (IU)	8.5	9.5	14	17.6
Vitamin B_1 (mg)	.03	.04	.06	.08
Vitamin B_2 (mg)	.04	.09	.08	.16
Niacin (mg)	2.28	2.38	5.66	4.03
Vitamin B_6 (mg)	.097	.085	.200	.167
Vitamin B_{12} (mg)	.316	.405	.455	.968
Folacin (mg)	.0038	.0042	.0064	.0086
Panthothenic (mg)	.199	.221	.387	.563
Vitamin C (mg)	.85	1.0	1.4	1.8
Vitamin D (mg)	16.1	12.2	15.2	22.9
Vitamin E (mg)	.55	.70	.95	.70
Calcium (mg)	21.6	12.1	50.1	34.2
Iodine (mg)	4.23	2.35	104	7.92
Iron (mg)	.68	.80	.98	1.45
Potassium (mg)	86.3	122	176	217
Magnesium (mg)	9.77	12.6	19.1	21.6
Sodium (mg)	302	207	558	566
Cholesterol (mg)	54.6	63	69.8	109

KENTUCKY FRIED CHICKEN CON'T.

	Keel	Mashed Potatoes	Gravy	Roll
Protein (g)	23.9	1.5	.4	1.8
Carbohydrate (g)	7.4	12.2	1.3	10.9
Fat (g)	12.3	.9	1.8	1.1
Vitamin A (IU)	19	18	3.0	5
Vitamin B$_1$ (mg)	.08	.01	.003	.10
Vitamin B$_2$ (mg)	.11	.02	.01	.04
Niacin (mg)	7.57	.76	.11	.98
Vitamin B$_6$ (mg)	.313	.110	.002	.014
Vitamin B$_{12}$ (mg)	.398	.063	.023	.022
Folacin (mg)	.0007	.0108	.0006	.0066
Panthothenic (mg)	.540	.212	.016	.071
Vitamin C (mg)	1.9	4.9	.15	.25
Vitamin D (mg)	7.20	7	3.8	3.2
Vitamin E (mg)	.96	.44	.12	.17
Calcium (mg)	29.8	15.6	1.69	21.3
Iodine (mg)	7.58	5.95	.85	14.6
Iron (mg)	1.17	.46	.13	.53
Potassium (mg)	267	232	8.29	28.6
Magnesium (mg)	27.7	14.9	.851	5.89
Sodium (mg)	631	268	57.1	118
Cholesterol (mg)	86.7	.20	.44	.64

KENTUCKY FRIED CHICKEN CON'T.

	Corn	Cole Slaw	Combination Dinner
Protein (g)	4.6	.9	32.6
Carbohydrates (g)	31.2	12.7	47.8
Fat (g)	2.8	7.5	37.8
Vitamin A (IU)	162	255	255
Vitamin B_1 (mg)	.12	.03	.24
Vitamin B_2 (mg)	.07	.02	.27
Niacin (mg)	1.20	.19	8.36
Vitamin B_6 (mg)	.207	.081	.471
Vitamin B_{12} (mg)	.111	.046	1.44
Folacin (mg)	.067	.0109	.0413
Panthothenic (mg)	.243	0.1	1.06
Vitamin C (mg)	2.6	31.7	36.6
Vitamin D (mg)	21.6	7.3	36.6
Vitamin E (mg)	1.21	1.53	3.51
Calcium (mg)	6.14	31.8	126
Iodine (mg)	6.8	4.6	33.9
Iron (mg)	.76	.53	3.78
Potassium (mg)	305	132	684
Magnesium (mg)	50.9	10.6	63.6
Sodium (mg)	11.1	225	1536
Cholesterol (mg)	.14	7.18	172

LONG JOHN SILVER'S

	Protein (grams)	Fat	Carbohydrates
Fish w/batter 2 pieces	21.6	21.6	21.4
Fish w/batter 3 pieces	32.4	32.4	32.1
Treasure Chest	30.2	32.7	31.6
Chicken Planks	27.2	23.2	34.7
Pag Legs	21.5	27.8	25.5
Ocean Scallops	11	13.4	29.5
Shrimp w/batter	8.4	12.6	30.4
Breaded Oysters	13.4	19.3	53.2
Breaded Clams	17.6	33.5	61.3
Fish Sandwich	21.8	30.7	49.4
French Fries	3.8	15.6	33.2
Cole Slaw	1.0	8	15.6
Corn on the Cob	5	3.5	28.7
Hush Puppies	2.7	6.6	20.3
Clam Chowder	4.5	3.3	14.9

McDONALD'S

	Apple Pie	Big Mac	Cheeseburger	Cherry Pie	Chocolate Shake
Protein (g)	1.87	25.7	15.1	2.0	9.9
Carbohydrates (g)	29.3	40.6	29.8	32.1	65.5
Fat (g)	14.3	33.	14.1	13.6	9.
Vitamin A (IU)	34.	530	345	114	349
Vitamin B_1 (mg)	.017	.388	.253	.026	.116
Vitamin B_2 (mg)	.187	.367	.23	.020	.436
Vitamin B_6 (mg)	.020	.265	.115	.022	134
Vitamin B_{12} (mg)	.034	1.8	.908	.035	1.16
Vitamin C (mg)	.85	2.24	1.61	.88	2.91
Vitamin D (mg)	1.7	32.64	12.6	1.76	43.6
Calcium (mg)	13.9	157	132	11.9	320
Copper (mg)	.048	.182	.108	.059	.186
Iron (mg)	.62	3.98	2.41	.59	.844
Magnesium (mg)	6.35	38.4	22.9	6.51	48.9
Phosphorus (mg)	27.4	314	205	27.2	335
Sodium (mg)	398	1010	767	427	300
Zinc (mg)	.162	4.69	2.6	.15	1.4
Cholesterol (mg)	12.4	85.7	37.3	13.4	29.7
Panthothenic (mg)	.212	.286	.333	.272	.640

	Egg McMuffin	English Muffin	Filet of Fish	French Fries	Hamburger
Protein (g)	18.5	5	14.3	3	12.3
Carbohydrates (g)	31	29.5	37.4	26.1	29.5
Fat (g)	14.8	5.3	25	11.5	9.8
Vitamin A (IU)	96.6	164	42	17	82
Vitamin B_1 (mg)	.469	.284	.264	122	.245
Vitamin B_2 (mg)	.442	.491	.195	.02	.184
Vitamin B_6 (mg)	.211	.044	.095	.218	.122
Vitamin B_{12} (mg)	745	.020	.82	.027	.806
Vitamin C (mg)	1.38	.819	1.39	12.53	1.73
Vitamin D (mg)	45.54	13.86	25	.88	12.24
Calcium (mg)	226	117	93.1	9.11	51
Copper (mg)	.119	.687	.097	.031	.099
Iron (mg)	2.93	1.51	1.71	.605	2.25
Magnesium (mg)	25.8	13	26.8	26.7	19.4
Phosphorus (mg)	322	74.3	229	101	126
Sodium (mg)	885	318	781	109	520
Zinc (mg)	1.92	.498	.89	.32	2.09
Cholesterol (mg)	229	12.6	47.3	8.57	24.5
Panthothenic (mg)	.773	.139	.222	.272	.296

McDONALD'S CONTINUED

	Hot Cakes	McDonald Cookies	Quarter Pounder	Quar. P. w/Cheese
Protein (g)	7.9	4.2	24.4	29.9
Carbohydrates (g)	93.9	48.7	32.7	32.2
Fat (g)	10.3	10.8	21.7	30.7
Vitamin A (IU)	257	26.8	133	660
Vitamin B_1 (mg)	.257	.228	.315	.31
Vitamin B_2 (mg)	.364	.234	.282	.369
Vitamin B_6 (mg)	.116	.028	1.88	.233
Vitamin B_{12} (mg)	.19	.034	2.66	2.15
Vitamin C (mg)	4.71	.938	1.7	2.72
Vitamin D (mg)	5.14	10	23.2	25.2
Calcium (mg)	103	11.6	63.1	219
Copper (mg)	.107	.068	.169	.175
Iron (mg)	2.23	1.47	4.1	4.29
Magnesium (mg)	28.20	10.8	37	40.7
Phosphorus (mg)	501	74.4	249	382
Sodium (mg)	1070	358	735	1236
Zinc (mg)	.685	.335	5.11	5.7
Cholesterol (mg)	47.1	10.2	67.1	95.6
Panthothenic (mg)	.235	.1	.531	.601

PIZZA HUT

	Standard Cheese	Standard Pepperoni	S. Pork/Mushroom	Super Supreme
Thin and Crispy				
Protein (g)	10	10	11	14.5
Carbohydrate (g)	22.5	22.5	20	25
Fat (g)	5.5	8	8	12
Thick and Chewy				
Protein (g)	12	12.5	13.5	17
Carbohydrate (g)	27.5	25	27.5	27.5
Fat (g)	5.5	8.2	7	13.5

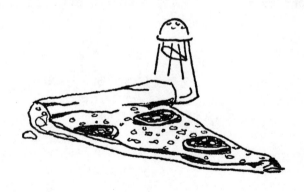

PIZZA HUT CON'T.

	Superstyle Cheese	Superstyle Pepperoni	S.s Pork/Mushroom	Supreme
Thin and Crispy				
Protein (g)	12.5	12	13.5	11
Carbohydrate (g)	25	22.5	22.5	25
Fat (g)	7	8.2	9.5	8
Thick and Chewy				
Protein (g)	15.6	14.5	14.5	14.5
Carbohydrate (g)	27.5	25	25	25
Fat (g)	7	9.5	9.5	9.5

PONDEROSA

Entree	Chopped Beef	Double Deluxe	Extra-cut Prime Rib	Extra-cut Ribeye	Fillet of Sole - Dinner
Protein (g)	40.6	45.4	47.9	41	29.8
Carbohydrate (g)					8.8
Fat (g)	16.7	18.8	22.7	20	9.8
Vitamin A (IU)	29.6	33.2	40	34.7	
Vitamin B_1 (mg)	0.1	0.1	0.1	0.1	0.1
Vitamin B_2 (mg)	0.3	0.4	0.4	0.3	0.1
Niacin (mg)	8.9	9.9	8.7	7.5	4.6
Vitamin B_6 (mg)	0.0	0.7	0.7	0.6	
Vitamin B_{12} (mg)		3	3	2.7	0.0
Folacin (mg)					
Panthothenic (mg)		1	1	0.9	
Vitamin C (mg)					
Vitamin D (mg)					
Vitamin E (mg)	0.6	0.2	0.2	0.2	
Calcium (mg)	17.8	19.8	20	17.3	35
Iodine (mg)	25.9	29	29.6	25.6	90.7
Iron (mg)	5.2	5.8	6.2	5.3	1
Potassium (mg)	460	924	536.5	464	462
Magnesium (mg)	31	35.2	38	32	36.4
Sodium (mg)	89	99.1	100.6	532.3	92.8
Cholesterol (mg)	103.6	115.8	118.1	147	118

126

PONDEROSA CON'T.

Entree	Fillet of Sole - Sandwich	Junior Patty	Prime Rib	Rib Eye	Rib Eye/Shrimp
Protein (g)	14.9	12.1	33.5	30.3	42.8
Carbohydrate (g)	4.4				6.2
Fat (g)	4.9	5.1	15.9	14.4	21.1
Vitamin A (IU)		8.9	28	25.3	57.4
Vitamin B$_1$ (mg)			0.1	0.1	0.1
Vitamin B$_2$ (mg)	0.1	0.1	0.3	0.2	0.4
Niacin (mg)	2.3	2.7	6.1	5.5	6.5
Vitamin B$_6$ (mg)		0.2	0.5	0.5	0.5
Vitamin B$_{12}$ (mg)		0.8	2.1	1.9	2.5
Folacin (mg)					
Panthothenic (mg)		0.3	0.7	0.7	0.8
Vitamin C (mg)					
Vitamin D (mg)					
Vitamin E (mg)		0.1	0.2	0.1	0.5
Calcium (mg)	17.5	5.4	14	12.7	97.6
Iodine (mg)	45.4	7.8	20.7	18.7	51.7
Iron (mg)	0.5	1.6	4.3	3.9	4.3
Potassium (mg)	231	259	375.2	339	479.8
Magnesium (mg)	18.3	9.8	26.6	34	65.4
Sodium (mg)	46.4	26.9	70.6	356.8	471.2
Cholesterol (mg)	59	31.4	82.6	74.2	151.2

PONDEROSA CON'T.

Entree	Shrimp	Steakhouse Deluxe	Strip Sirloin	Super Sirloin	T-Bone
Protein (g)	19.9	22.7	42.8	59.1	58.5
Carbohydrate (g)	9.8				
Fat (g)	10.6	9.4	10.3	14.2	13.7
Vitamin A (IU)	51	16.6	18.3	25.3	18.8
Vitamin B$_1$ (mg)	0.1	0.1	0.1	0.2	0.2
Vitamin B$_2$ (mg)	0.3	0.2	0.3	0.8	0.5
Niacin (mg)	1.6	5	8.5	11.7	11.3
Vitamin B$_6$ (mg)	0.1	0.4	0.6	0.8	0.8
Vitamin B$_{12}$ (mg)	0.9	1.5	2.4	3.3	3.4
Folacin (mg)					
Panthothenic (mg)	0.3	0.5	0.8	1.1	1.2
Vitamin C (mg)					
Vitamin D (mg)					
Vitamin E (mg)	0.6	0.1	0.2	0.2	0.2
Calcium (mg)	125	9.9	17.1	23.6	22.6
Iodine (mg)	53	14.5	23.2	32	32.9
Iron (mg)	0.6	2.9	5.1	7.1	7
Potassium (mg)	224	462	481	663.8	809.6
Magnesium (mg)	50	17.6	28	38.2	38.4
Sodium (mg)	182	49.8	523.9	695.2	850.6
Cholesterol (mg)	122.5	57.9	92.7	128	131.6

PONDEROSA CON'T.

	Chopped Beef	Double Deluxe	Extra-cut Prime Rib	Extra-cut Rib Eye	Fillet of Sole Dinner
Dinner					
Protein (g)	51.9	55.6	59.2	52.3	41.1
Carbohydrate (g)	73.5	67.2	73.5	73.5	82.3
Fat (g)	24.8	33	30.8	28.1	17.9
Vitamin A (IU)	1913.6	409	1924	1918	1884
Vitamin B$_1$ (mg)	0.6	0.5	0.6	0.5	0.5
Vitamin B$_2$ (mg)	0.6	0.6	0.6	0.6	0.4
Niacin (mg)	13.9	14.5	13.7	12.5	9.6
Vitamin B$_6$ (mg)	0.8	0.9	1.5	1.4	0.8
Vitamin B$_{12}$ (mg)		3	3	2.7	
Folacin (mg)	0.1			0.1	
Panthothenic (mg)	0.5	1.8	1.5	1.4	0.5
Vitamin C (mg)	61.7	25.2	61.7	61.7	61.7
Vitamin D (mg)					
Vitamin E (mg)	1.1	0.6	0.8	0.7	0.6
Calcium (mg)	123.1	93.5	125.8	123.1	140.8
Iodine (mg)	144.4	70.5	147.4	143.4	208.5
Iron (mg)	9.7	8.8	10.7	9.8	5.5
Potassium (mg)	1783	1840	1859.5	1787	1785
Magnesium (mg)	78.2	66.7	85.2	79.2	84.6
Sodium (mg)	466.6	719	478.2	900.9	470.4
Cholesterol (mg)	116.1	115.8	130.6	159.5	130.5

PONDEROSA CON'T.

	Fillet of Sole Sandwich	Junior Patty	Prime Rib	Rib Eye	Rib Eye/Shrimp
Dinner					
Protein (g)	24.8	19.2	44.8	41.6	54.1
Carbohydrate (g)	72.3	51.2	73.5	73.5	79.7
Fat (g)	19.1	17.9	24	22.5	29.2
Vitamin A (IU)	7.5	8.9	1912	1909.3	1941.4
Vitamin B_1 (mg)	0.4	0.3	0.5	0.5	1.3
Vitamin B_2 (mg)	0.3	0.3	0.5	0.5	0.6
Niacin (mg)	6.8	6.4	0.5	10.5	11.5
Vitamin B_6 (mg)	0.2	0.4	1.3	1.2	1.3
Vitamin B_{12} (mg)		0.8	2.1	1.9	2.5
Folacin (mg)					
Panthothenic (mg)	0.8	0.9	1.2	1.2	1.3
Vitamin C (mg)	35.8	16.8	61.7	61.7	61.7
Vitamin D (mg)					
Vitamin E (mg)	0.3	0.3	0.7	0.7	1.1
Calcium (mg)	93.8	68	119.8	118.5	203.4
Iodine (mg)	76	35.4	138.5	136.5	169.5
Iron (mg)	3.2	3.7	8.8	8.4	8.8
Potassium (mg)	1046.5	1004	1698.2	1162.1	1802.8
Magnesium (mg)	42.4	24.1	73.8	81.2	112.6
Sodium (mg)	386	228.7	448.2	734.4	848.2
Cholesterol (mg)	59	31.4	95.1	86.7	163.7

PONDEROSA CON'T.

	Shrimp	Steakhouse Deluxe	Strip Sirloin	Super Sirloin	T-Bone
Dinner					
Protein (g)	31.2	32.9	54.1	70.4	69.8
Carbohydrate (g)	83.3	67.2	73.5	73.5	73.5
Fat (g)	18.7	23.5	18.4	22.3	21.8
Vitamin A (IU)	1935	392.4	1898.3	1909.3	1902.8
Vitamin B$_1$ (mg)	0.5	0.4	0.6	0.6	0.6
Vitamin B$_2$ (mg)	0.5	0.4	0.6	0.7	0.7
Niacin (mg)	6.6	9.6	13.5	16.7	16.3
Vitamin B$_6$ (mg)	0.9	0.6	1.4	1.6	1.6
Vitamin B$_{12}$ (mg)	0.9	1.5	2.4	3.3	3.4
Folacin (mg)				0.1	0.1
Panthothenic (mg)	0.8	1.3	1.3	1.6	1.7
Vitamin C (mg)	61.7	25.2	61.7	61.7	61.7
Vitamin D (mg)					
Vitamin E (mg)	1.1	0.6	0.7	0.8	0.8
Calcium (mg)	240.8	83.6	122.9	129.4	128.4
Iodine (mg)	170.8	56	141	149.8	150.7
Iron (mg)	5.1	6	9.6	11.6	11.5
Potassium (mg)	1547	1378.1	1804	1986.8	2132.6
Magnesium (mg)	97.2	49.1	75.2	85.4	85.6
Sodium (mg)	559.6	669.7	901.5	1072.8	1228.2
Cholesterol (mg)	135	57.9	105.2	140.5	144.1

PONDEROSA CON'T.

	Coca-Cola	Coffee	Dr. Pepper	Milk
Beverage				
Protein (g)				8.5
Carbohydrate (g)	24		24.8	14.8
Fat (g)				8.5
Vitamin A (IU)				350
Vitamin B_1 (mg)				0.1
Vitamin B_2 (mg)				0.4
Niacin (mg)		0.5		0.2
Vitamin B_6 (mg)				0.1
Vitamin B_{12} (mg)				1
Folacin (mg)				
Panthothenic (mg)				0.8
Vitamin C (mg)				2
Vitamin D (mg)				100
Vitamin E (mg)				0.1
Calcium (mg)		4	6.4	288
Iodine (mg)				33.9
Iron (mg)		0.2		0.1
Potassium (mg)	88	65	1.6	351
Magnesium (mg)				31.7
Sodium (mg)	20	2	18.4	122
Cholesterol (mg)				26.8

PONDEROSA CON'T.

Beverage	Rootbeer	Sprite	Tab	Tea
Protein (g)				
Carbohydrate (g)	25.6	24	1	
Fat (g)				
Vitamin A (IU)				
Vitamin B1 (mg)				
Vitamin B2 (mg)				
Niacin (mg)				0.1
Vitamin B6 (mg)				
Vitamin B12 (mg)				
Folacin (mg)				
Panthothenic (mg)				
Vitamin C (mg)				
Vitamin D (mg)				
Vitamin E (mg)				
Calcium (mg)				5
Iodine (mg)				
Iron (mg)				0.2
Potassium (mg)				
Magnesium (mg)				
Sodium (mg)		42	30	
Cholesterol (mg)				

133

PONDEROSA CON'T.

	Baked Potato	Butter	Catsup	Cocktail Sauce	Dill Pickles
Miscellaneous					
Protein (g)	4		0.3	1.1	0.2
Carbohydrate (g)	32.8		4.3	14.5	0.5
Fat (g)	0.2	4.1	0.1	0.3	
Vitamin A (IU)		165	240	768	15
Vitamin B$_1$ (mg)	0.2				
Vitamin B$_2$ (mg)	0.1				
Niacin (mg)	2.7		0.3	1	
Vitamin B$_6$ (mg)	0.5	0.2			
Vitamin B$_{12}$ (mg)					
Folacin (mg)					
Panthothenic (mg)					
Vitamin C (mg)	31		3	10	1.5
Vitamin D (mg)					
Vitamin E (mg)	0.1	0.1			
Calcium (mg)	14	1	4	17	4.5
Iodine (mg)	56.6	0.7			
Iron (mg)	1.1		0.1	0.4	0.2
Potassium (mg)	782	1	62	220	39
Magnesium (mg)			4	12.8	2.3
Sodium (mg)	6	49	177	143	279
Cholesterol (mg)		12.5			

PONDEROSA CON'T.

	French Fries	Kaiser Roll	Lemon Wedge	Lettuce - 0.5 oz.	Lettuce - 3 oz.
Miscellaneous					
Protein (g)	3.6	5	0.3	0.2	1
Carbohydrate (g)	30.2	33	2.7	0.4	2.1
Fat (g)	11.1	3.4	0.1		0.2
Vitamin A (IU)			7.5	135.8	815
Vitamin B$_1$ (mg)	0.1				0.1
Vitamin B$_2$ (mg)	0.1				0.1
Niacin (mg)	2.6	1.3	0.1		0.3
Vitamin B$_6$ (mg)	0.2	0.2			0.1
Vitamin B$_{12}$ (mg)		0.1			
Folacin (mg)					
Panthothenic (mg)	0.5				0.2
Vitamin C (mg)	16.8			1.1	6.7
Vitamin D (mg)					
Vitamin E (mg)	0.2				0.1
Calcium (mg)	12.6	45.4	15.3	4.9	29.4
Iodine (mg)	23.5	6.5		3.9	23.5
Iron (mg)	1.2	1.1	0.2	0.3	1.7
Potassium (mg)	717.6	58	36.3	36.9	222
Magnesium (mg)		23		1.5	9.2
Sodium (mg)	4.8	311	0.8	1.3	7.6
Cholesterol (mg)					

PONDEROSA CON'T.

	Margarine	Mayonnaise	Mustard	Onion	Blue Cheese Salad Dressing
Miscellaneous					
Protein (g)		0.2	0.2	0.2	0.7
Carbohydrate (g)		0.3	0.3	0.9	0.9
Fat (g)	4.1	11.2	0.2		5.6
Vitamin A (IU)	165	40		4	40
Vitamin B_1 (mg)					
Vitamin B_2 (mg)					
Niacin (mg)					
Vitamin B_6 (mg)					
Vitamin B_{12} (mg)					
Folacin (mg)					
Panthothenic (mg)					
Vitamin C (mg)				1	
Vitamin D (mg)					
Vitamin E (mg)					
Calcium (mg)	1	3	4	3	11
Iodine (mg)	0.7		0.1	3.1	
Iron (mg)		0.1	0.1	0.1	
Potassium (mg)	1	5	7	16	3
Magnesium (mg)				1	
Sodium (mg)	49	84	63	1	115
Cholesterol (mg)					

PONDEROSA CON'T.

	Creamy Italian Salad Dressing	French Salad Dressing	Oil/Vinegar Salad Dressing	1000 Island Salad Dressing	Steak Sauce
Miscellaneous					
Protein (g)				0.1	0.2
Carbohydrate (g)	1.2	4	0.4	2.9	2
Fat (g)	6.1	4.7	6	4.6	0.2
Vitamin A (IU)		32		30	62
Vitamin B$_1$ (mg)					
Vitamin B$_2$ (mg)					
Niacin (mg)					
Vitamin B$_6$ (mg)					
Vitamin B$_{12}$ (mg)					
Folacin (mg)					
Panthothenic (mg)					
Vitamin C (mg)					
Vitamin D (mg)					
Vitamin E (mg)					
Calcium (mg)	3.1	3.2	0.5	2.5	3
Iodine (mg)					
Iron (mg)		0.2		0.1	0.1
Potassium (mg)	3.3	10.4	7	6.5	30
Magnesium (mg)					
Sodium (mg)	182	148	0.1	74	143
Cholesterol (mg)					

137

PONDEROSA CON'T.

	Steakhouse Deluxe Bun	Tartar Sauce	Tomato - small	Tomato - 2 slices
Miscellaneous				
Protein (g)	6	0.2	1.1	0.3
Carbohydrate (g)	35	1.5	4.7	1.2
Fat (g)	3	10	0.2	0.1
Vitamin A (IU)		55	900	225
Vitamin B$_1$ (mg)	0.2		0.1	
Vitamin B$_2$ (mg)	0.1			
Niacin (mg)	1.8		0.7	0.2
Vitamin B$_6$ (mg)			0.1	
Vitamin B$_{12}$ (mg)				
Folacin (mg)				
Panthothenic (mg)	0.3		0.3	0.1
Vitamin C (mg)		1	23	5.8
Vitamin D (mg)				
Vitamin E (mg)	0.1		0.4	0.1
Calcium (mg)	48.4	4	13	3.3
Iodine (mg)	7.1		27.4	7
Iron (mg)	1.3	0.2	0.5	0.1
Potassium (mg)	61.6		244	61
Magnesium (mg)	24.2		14	3.5
Sodium (mg)	334		3	0.8
Cholesterol (mg)				

POPPIN' FRESH

	Protein	Carbohydrate	Fat
Chef's Salad	48	25	57
Custard Pie	8	45	19
Dairy Salad	43	28	38
Dinner Salad	4	13	20
Doughboy Salad	9	26	43
Pumpkin Pie	6	57	15
Shrimp Salad	28	22	49
Tuna Salad	24	35	45

RED LOBSTER

	Carbohydrate (g)	Fat (g)
Entree		
Albacore Tuna	0.2	0.7 - 18.2
Breaded Fried Pollock/Whitefish	6.5	8.9
Catfish	0.2	0.3 - 11.0
Chicken, Fried	3.7	19.3 - 22.5
Clams	1.7	1.4 - 2.5
Cod	1.0	0.1 - 1.0
Crab, Snow	1.0	1.9
Egg	9.7	0.2
Flounder	0.6	0.1 - 2.5
Garlic Bread	18.7	5.1
Grouper	1.0	0.2 - 2.3
Haddock	0.6	0.1 - 1.2
Halibut	0.0	0.7 - 5.2
Hamburger Pattie	0.0	21.2
Hush Puppies	29.1	14.4
Lobster	0.8	0.6 - 1.9
Oysters	4.4	0.7 - 2.6
Perch	0.0	0.3 - 1.5
Pollock	0.0	0.6 - 1.4
Potato	17.0	0.1
Scallops	3.3	0.3

RED LOBSTER CON'T.

	Carbohydrate (g)	Fat (g)
Shrimp	3.3	0.1 - 3.2
Sirloin Steak	0.0	27.5
Snapper	0.5	0.4 - 7.4
Sole	0.6	0.2 - 1.7
Tuna, Other	0.1	0.1 - 9.5
Turbot	0.2	2.9
Walleyed Pike	0.5	0.8 - 1.9
Whiting	0.0	1.0 - 3.0
Broiled Fisherman's Platter	80.5	42.8
Broiled Stuffed Flounder	70.4	45.1
Mariner's Platter	78.7	42.1
Sampler Platter	66.9	31.7
Shore Platter	76.6	38.6
Steak and Lobster	59.3	104.3

STEAK N SHAKE

	Baked Beans	Baked Ham Sand.	Chili	Chili Mac	Chili - Three Ways
Protein (g)	8.6	28.9	15.9	14.5	18.9
Carbohydrate (g)	26.9	36.5	36.9	34.5	44.6
Fat (g)	3.7	22	14.1	12.4	16
Vitamin A (IU)	184.1	189.7	112.8	979	1333.4
Vitamin B$_1$ (mg)	0.1	0.5	0.1	0.1	0.2
Vitamin B$_2$ (mg)		0.3	0.1	0.2	0.3
Niacin (mg)	0.9	1.1	2.6	2.2	3
Vitamin C (mg)	2.8	1.2		4.6	6.4
Calcium (mg)	76.5	72.6	66.6	122.3	140.9
Iron (mg)	2.6	3.7	3.5	3.2	4.3
Phosphorus (mg)	130.3	305.9	254.5	162.7	202.5
Potassium (mg)	297.4	417.4	453.8	247.6	334.4
Sodium (mg)	655.6	1858.3	1156.7	1301.7	1734.1
Ash (g)	2.3	3.2	4	4.4	5.8
Fiber (g)	2	0.2	1.2	0.3	0.4

STEAK N SHAKE CON'T.

	Cottage Cheese	Egg Sand.	French Fries	Ham/Egg Sand.	Lettuce
Protein (g)	11.9	11.8	3.3	35.7	1
Carbohydrate (g)	2.9	33.4	27.7	33.3	6.9
Fat (g)	3.6	9.9	10.2	17.2	15.3
Vitamin A (IU)	291.7	673.3		668.2	722
Vitamin B$_1$ (mg)		0.1	0.1	0.5	
Vitamin B$_2$ (mg)	2.2	0.2	0.1	0.4	
Niacin (mg)	0.1	0.8	2.4	1.1	0.3
Vitamin C (mg)	1.2	0.3	16.2		9.4
Calcium (mg)	86.1	82.3	11.6	90.9	21.9
Iron (mg)	0.6	1.6	1	4.5	1.2
Phosphorus (mg)	131.1	162.3	85.5	399.2	12
Potassium (mg)	112.7	139.7	664.5	433.5	224.9
Sodium (mg)	198.2	490	297.2	1849.8	223.2
Ash (g)	1	2.1	1.4	3.4	1.1
Fiber (g)	0.1		0.8	0.1	0.4

STEAK N SHAKE CON'T.

	Low Calorie Platter	Steakburger	Steakburger W/Cheese	Super Steakburger
Protein (g)	36.6	18.1	22.8	30.4
Carbohydrate (g)	3.3	33.3	33.7	33.3
Fat (g)	13.7	7.1	13.3	12.1
Vitamin A (IU)	402.4	16.4	262.4	25.4
Vitamin B$_1$ (mg)	0.1	0.1	0.1	0.1
Vitamin B$_2$ (mg)	2.4	0.2	1	0.3
Niacin (mg)	0.8	1	1	1.3
Vitamin C (mg)	3.6	0.7	0.7	0.7
Calcium (mg)	98.3	62.6	205.5	68
Iron (mg)	3.6	2	2.2	3.5
Phosphorus (mg)	340.9	169.2	327.3	272.7
Potassium (mg)	650.3	335.4	351.8	586.5
Sodium (mg)	241.5	424.9	657.8	446.6
Ash (g)	2.3	2.1	3.1	2.7
Fiber (g)	0.1	0.2	0.2	0.2

STEAK N SHAKE CON'T.

	Super Steakburger w/cheese	Triple Steakburger	Triple Steakburger w/cheese	Toasted Cheese
Protein (g)	35.1	42.7	52.1	8.7
Carbohydrate (g)	33.7	33.3	34.1	23.5
Fat (g)	18.3	17.1	29.5	13.3
Vitamin A (IU)	271.4	34.4	526.4	482.1
Vitamin B_1 (mg)	0.1	0.2	0.2	
Vitamin B_2 (mg)	1.1	0.4	2	0.9
Niacin (mg)	1.3	1.5	1.5	0.5
Vitamin C (mg)	0.7	0.7	0.7	0.5
Calcium (mg)	210.9	73.4	359.2	184
Iron (mg)	3.7	5	5.4	0.3
Phosphorus (mg)	430.8	376.2	692.4	204.5
Potassium (mg)	602.9	837.6	870.4	76
Sodium (mg)	679.4	468.1	933.9	606
Ash (g)	3.7	3.4	5.4	2.3
Fiber (g)	0.2	0.2	0.2	0.1

STEAK N SHAKE CON'T.

	Apple Danish	Apple Pie	Brownie	Brownie Fudge Sundae	Cheese Cake
Miscellaneous					
Protein (g)	5.7	3.5	3.2	6.6	6.4
Carbohydrate (g)	35.2	60.6	39.1	80.6	60.9
Fat (g)	23.8	17.7	11.5	35.2	11.1
Vitamin A (IU)	470.3	47.7	112	924.7	151.2
Vitamin B$_1$ (mg)	0.1			0.1	0.2
Vitamin B$_2$ (mg)	0.2	0.1	0.4	0.2	
Niacin (mg)	0.6	6.4	0.1	0.4	0.4
Vitamin C (mg)		1.6		1.2	15.1
Calcium (mg)	40	12.7	49	240.1	92
Iron (mg)	0.7	0.5	0.7	1.4	1.5
Phosphorus (mg)	85.2	35	91.7	268.4	117.2
Potassium (mg)	88.1	127.2	107.8	404.2	117.2
Sodium (mg)	351.6	478.6	164.5	261.9	293.6
Ash (g)	1.3	1.6	0.9	2.4	1.4
Fiber (g)	0.1	0.6	0.2	0.4	3.8

STEAK N SHAKE CON'T.

	Cheese Cake w/strawberries	Cherry Pie	Cherry Pie ala Mode	Choc. Shake	Hot Fudge Nut Sundae
Protein (g)	6.8	5.5	5.8	12.7	185.7
Carbohydrate (g)	65.1	47.9	63.2	57.1	50.9
Fat (g)	11.4	13.8	21.6	37.8	34.4
Vitamin A (IU)	180.8	325	648.8	1271.4	1009.1
Vitamin B_1 (mg)	0.2		0.1	0.1	0.1
Vitamin B_2 (mg)	0.2	0.1	0.3	0.5	0.4
Niacin (mg)	0.4	0.3	0.3	0.2	0.4
Vitamin C (mg)	44.4		0.7	2.4	1.6
Calcium (mg)	102.5	93.8	201.3	412.5	244.9
Iron (mg)	2	1.1	1.2	0.3	1.4
Phosphorus (mg)	127.7	101.3	185.9	325	284.6
Potassium (mg)	198	118.8	252	514.6	415.9
Sodium (mg)	294.1	267.5	313.9	177.7	121
Ash (g)	1.6	1.6	2.2	2.6	2
Fiber (g)	4.3				0.3

STEAK N SHAKE CON'T.

	Ice Cream	Lemon Drink	Lemon Float	Lemon Freeze	Orange Drink
Protein (g)	0.5		17.5	14.9	
Carbohydrate (g)	22.9	22.3	81.8	68.5	21.6
Fat (g)	11.7		18.6	24.9	
Vitamin A (IU)	485.7		766.5	1043.8	18
Vitamin B$_1$ (mg)	0.1		0.2	0.2	
Vitamin B$_2$ (mg)	0.2		0.8	0.7	
Niacin (mg)	0.1		0.4	3.5	
Vitamin C (mg)	1.1		3.7	00.0	64.8
Calcium (mg)	161.2		569.4	488.9	
Iron (mg)	0.1		0.4	0.3	
Phosphorus (mg)	217	452.6	388		
Potassium (mg)	199.8		711.8	584.4	
Sodium (mg)	69.6		248.2	212.7	
Ash (g)		1	3.7	3.2	
Fiber (g)					

STEAK N SHAKE CON'T.

	Orange Float	Orange Freeze	Strawberry Shake	Strawberry Sundae	Vanilla Shake
Protein (g)	15.8	13.9	16.2	1.6	12.9
Carbohydrate (g)	73.9	62.8	61.5	29.3	58.4
Fat (g)	16.8	23.8	40	21.7	38.4
Vitamin A (IU)	693	999.7	1676	937	1610
Vitamin B_1 (mg)	0.2	1.4	0.1	0.1	0.1
Vitamin B_2 (mg)	0.7	0.7	0.6	0.3	0.6
Niacin (mg)	0.3	0.3	0.3	0.4	0.3
Vitamin C (mg)	3.3	3.3	3.3	30.9	3.2
Calcium (mg)	514.8	456	443.2	199.2	421
Iron (mg)	0.3	0.3	0.3	0.6	0.3
Phosphorus (mg)	409.2	362	349.2	159.1	331.9
Potassium (mg)	643.5	573	552.6	318.2	525.5
Sodium (mg)	224.4	198.4	190.9	81.4	181.4
Ash (g)	3.3	2.9	2.7	1.4	2.6
Fiber (g)				0.7	

TACO BELL

	Bean Burrito	Beef Burrito	Beefy Tostada	Bellbeefer
Protein (g)	11	30	19	15
Carbohydrate (g)	48	37	19	23
Fat (g)	12	21	12	7
Vitamin A (IU)	1657	1675	3450	2961
Vitamin B$_1$ (mg)	0.4	0.3	0.2	0.2
Vitamin B$_2$ (mg)	0.2	0.4	0.3	0.2
Niacin (mg)	2.2	7.0	3.3	3.7
Vitamin C (mg)	15.2	15.2	12.7	10
Calcium (mg)	98	83	208	40
Iron (mg)	2.8	4.6	3.4	2.6
Potassium (mg)	235	320	277	183
Phosphorus (mg)	173	288	265	140
Sodium (mg)	272	327	138	231

TACO BELL CON'T.

	Bellbeefer w/cheese	Burrito Supreme	Combo. Burrito	Enchirito
Protein (g)	19	21	21	25
Carbohydrate (g)	23	43	43	42
Fat (g)	12	22	16	21
Vitamin A (IU)	3146	3462	1666	1178
Vitamin B_1 (mg)	0.2	0.3	0.3	0.3
Vitamin B_2 (mg)	0.3	0.4	0.3	0.4
Niacin (mg)	3.7	4.7	4.6	4.7
Vitamin C (mg)	10	16	15.2	9.5
Calcium (mg)	147	121	91	259
Iron (mg)	2.7	3.8	3.7	3.8
Potassium (mg)	195	350	278	491
Phosphorus (mg)	208	245	230	338
Sodium (mg)	330	367	300	1175

TACO BELL CON'T.

	Pintos 'n Cheese	Taco	Tostada
Protein (g)	11	15	9
Carbohydrate (g)	21	14	25
Fat (g)	5	8	6
Vitamin A (IU)	3123	120	3152
Vitamin B$_1$ (mg)	0.3	0.1	0.2
Vitamin B$_2$ (mg)	0.2	0.2	0.2
Niacin (mg)	0.9	2.9	0.8
Vitamin C (mg)	9.3	0.2	9.7
Calcium (mg)	150	120	191
Iron (mg)	2.3	2.5	2.3
Potassium (mg)	307	143	172
Phosphorus (mg)	210	175	186
Sodium (mg)	102	79	101

TACO JOHN'S

	Taco	Soft Shell	Regular Burrito	Beefy Burrito
Protein (g)	25	34	35	59
Carbohydrates (g)	15.3	38.9	51.9	41.6
Fat (g)	9.4	10.4	7.2	20.3
Vitamin A (IU)	8	6	5	5
Vitamin B$_1$ (mg)	11	23	37	27
Vitamin B$_2$ (mg)	11	18	19	26
Niacin (mg)	16	25	19	40
Vitamin C (mg)	9	9	4	5
Calcium (mg)	7	8	17	14
Iron (mg)	13	21	25	31
Potassium (mg)	209	225	369	288
Sodium (mg)	131	140	197	240

TACO JOHN'S CONTINUED

	Combination Burrito	Taco Burger	Taco Bravo	Enchilada
Protein (g)	51	36	43	51
Carbohydrates (g)	48.5	32.4	53.4	30.9
Fat (g)	15.7	13.8	12.8	16.9
Vitamin A (IU)	5	6	11	9
Vitamin B_1 (mg)	34	20	33	28
Vitamin B_2 (mg)	24	18	20	20
Niacin (mg)	32	25	28	29
Vitamin C (mg)	4	9	13	9
Calcium (mg)	15	11	15	16
Iron (mg)	31	20	27	29
Potassium (mg)	364	247	356	450
Sodium (mg)	219	397	200	303

TACO JOHN'S CONTINUED

	Tostada	Beefy Tostada	Comb. Tostada	Chili
Protein (g)	23	24	17.9	19.9
Carbohydrates (g)	30.3	19.7	25	34.1
Fat (g)	5.5	18.3	11.7	14.2
Vitamin A (IU)	12	12	12	10
Vitamin B$_1$ (mg)	26	17	22	32
Vitamin B$_2$ (mg)	12	20	16	17
Niacin (mg)	7	30	18	18
Vitamin C (mg)	12	13	13	11
Calcium (mg)	17	14	15	18
Iron (mg)	17	23	20	26
Potassium (mg)	439	354	397	479
Sodium (mg)	141	228	185	395

WENDY'S

	Protein	Carbohydrates	Fat
Single Cheeseburger	33	34	34
Double Cheeseburger	50	41	48
Triple Cheeseburger	72	35	68
Chili	5	21	8
French Fries	5	41	16
Frosty	9	54	16
Single Hamburger	26	34	26
Double Hamburger	44	34	40
Triple Hamburger	72	35	68

WHITE CASTLE

	Bun	Cheeseburger	Fish without T. sauce	French Fries	Hamburger
Protein (g)	2.2	7.8	7.4	3.1	6
Carbohydrate (g)	12.36	17.6	20.2	27.4	17.5
Fat (g)	0.6	8.7	8.5	10.8	6.8
Sodium (mg)		1.7	1.1	0.8	1.7
Ash (g)	0.1	0.8	0.6	1.0	0.6
Fiber (g)	0.2	1.7	1.8	2	1.5
Moisture (mg)	7.0	31.0	27.8	32	24.5
Nitrogen Free Extract	12.2	16	18.3	25.4	16.0

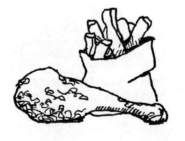